5 INGREDIENTS
QUICK & EASY FOOD

Food photography DAVID LOFTUS

Portrait photography PAUL STUART & JAMIE OLIVER

Design JAMES VERITY at SUPERFANTASTIC

MICHAEL JOSEPH
an imprint of
PENGUIN BOOKS

DEDICATED
TO MY FIVE
FAVOURITE
INGREDIENTS

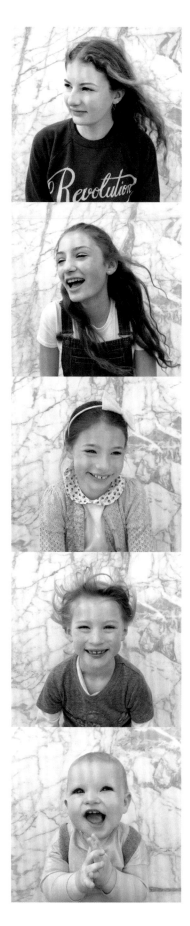

POPPY HONEY ROSIE

DAISY BOO PAMELA

PETAL BLOSSOM RAINBOW

BUDDY BEAR MAURICE

RIVER ROCKET BLUE DALLAS

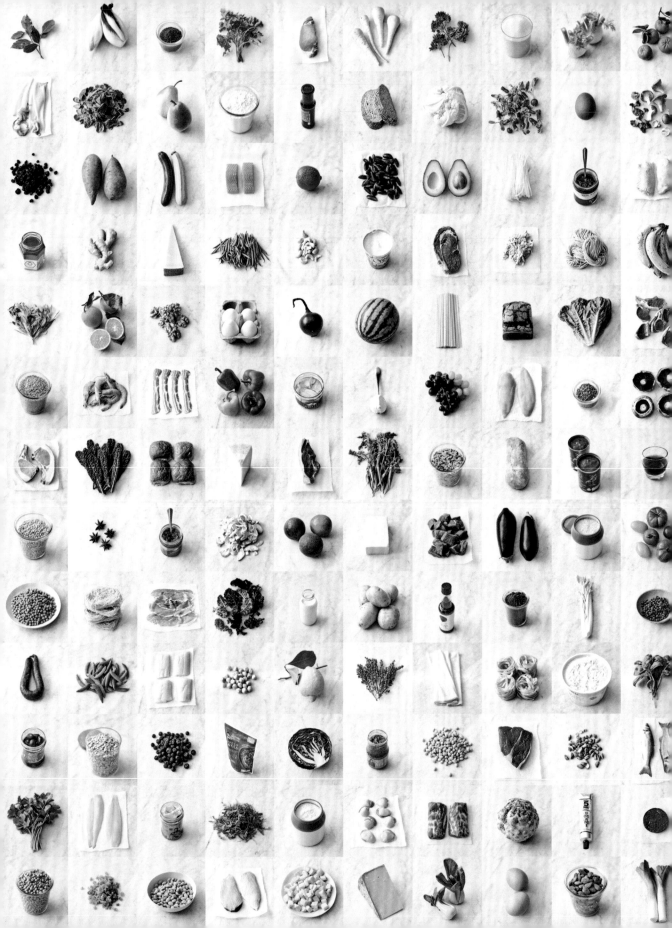

CONTENTS

5 INGREDIENTS

Quick & Easy Food focuses unapologetically on genius combinations of just five ingredients that work together to deliver an utterly delicious result, giving maximum flavour, with minimum fuss. These are dishes you can get on the table in 30 minutes or less; or that are ridiculously quick to put together with just 10 minutes hands-on time, while the oven or hob then does the rest of the work.

I want everyone to enjoy cooking from scratch and, armed with this book, there are no excuses. I've made it as simple as possible to cook amazing food, celebrating the joy of five ingredients, any day of the week, whatever the occasion – everything from a quick weeknight supper to a weekend feast with friends.

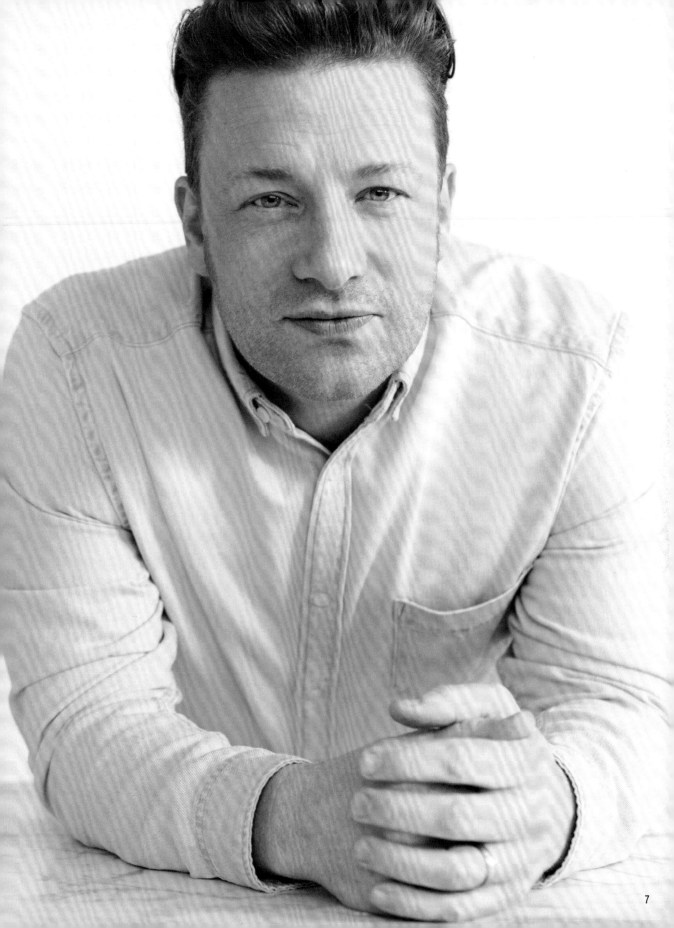

The concept is straightforward, but behind the scenes it's the structure, clever planning and spirit of the book – as well as relentless recipe testing – that's been the key to success. The creation of the recipes has ignited a real sense of excitement in me to wow people with brilliant combinations that are just crying out to be enjoyed. This is about empowerment and getting back to basics. The recipes are short, and I've included a visual ingredients key on every page to take you from business on one side to gastronomic delight on the other, where you see those tempting, finished dishes.

Looking at the contents, you'll see that I've tried to cover all the bases: fabulous ways with proteins; bigging up brilliant veg; making salads exciting; creating stress-free, tasty fish dishes; celebrating humble pasta; and helping you kick your rice and noodle game into action. Plus, a bonus bumper chapter of delightful sweet treats, easy puds and simple biscuits you can enjoy with a good cup of tea. I'm presuming you have a pantry store you can call on, but these lists are often too long, so I've kept the pantry for this book super-simple at – you guessed it – just five key ingredients (see page 10 for details).

INSTANT INSPIRATION & BAGS OF IDEAS

With the exception of the sweet treats chapter, 70% of the recipes are healthy and I've included nutrition info on every page, should you wish to use it. Not every recipe gives you a balanced meal – some are simply brilliant ways of cooking a piece of meat or fish that will blow your mind, combos that elevate veg to a whole new level, beautiful, bright salads that help you to up your veg and fruit intake, as well as elements you can mix, match and bolster however you like. The important thing to remember is to get your balance right across the week – refresh your memory on pages 304 and 305.

Food content is shared in such a variety of ways now, from Pinterest, BuzzFeed and YouTube to word of mouth and everything in between, all of it giving you great tricks, hacks and nuggets of info that are easy to digest, as well as enticing visual references. My intention with this book was to bottle all of that and make sense of it in one place, sharing solid, exciting recipes that by their very nature are based on clever tips, tricks and techniques. I've got straight to the point and kept things super-simple, so that you can flick through these pages and get instant inspiration and bags of ideas. I hope you enjoy it, and that you feel it's a book you want to share with friends, family, kids off to uni, you name it.

SO GUYS, HAPPY COOKING, AND PLEASE SHARE YOUR
FINISHED DISHES ON INSTAGRAM #QUICKANDEASYFOOD

I've kept this to just five ingredients that I consider to be everyday staples. Cooking is simply impossible without these items at your fingertips, and I believe every household should have them in stock. Even though my own pantry is packed full of all sorts of things, it's these five that you'll see popping up regularly throughout the book and that you need in order to cook any of the recipes. They aren't included in each individual ingredients list as I'm presuming that you'll stock up before you start cooking. The five heroes are **olive oil** for cooking, **extra virgin olive oil** for dressing and finishing dishes, **red wine vinegar** as a good all-rounder when it comes to acidity and balancing marinades, sauces and dressings, and, of course, **sea salt** and **black pepper** for seasoning. Get these and you're away!

QUALITY NOT QUANTITY

As is always the case in cooking, but especially in this book, the success of the recipes comes down to you buying the best-quality ingredients you can get your hands on. As you haven't got loads of stuff to buy for each recipe, I'm hoping it will give you even more of an excuse to trade up where you can, buying the best meats, fish or veggies you can find. To this end, remember that shopping in season always allows your food to be more nutritious, more delicious and more affordable.

Ingredients that noticeably make a difference on the flavour front when you choose best quality are: chorizo, sausages, black pudding, smoked salmon, jarred tuna, jarred beans and chickpeas, tinned plum tomatoes, ice cream and dark chocolate.

THE FREEZER IS YOUR FRIEND

I've designed a lot of the recipes to serve two, so that it's easy to scale up or down as you need to. Some recipes are more naturally suited to being made in bigger quantities, particularly when it comes to slow cooking, but you can always freeze extra portions for another day. Just remember to let food cool before freezing, breaking it down into portions so it cools quicker and you can get it into the freezer within 2 hours of cooking. Make sure everything is well wrapped, meat and fish especially, and labelled up for future reference. Thaw in the fridge before use. Generally, if you've frozen cooked food, don't freeze it again after you've reheated it.

CELEBRATING CONDIMENTS

I use a lot of condiments in this book, like mango chutney, curry pastes, black bean and teriyaki sauces, miso and pesto. These are items you can find in all supermarkets, of an extraordinary quality, these days. They guarantee flavour and save hours of time in preparation, as well as saving on cupboard space and food waste. For quick and easy meals, these products are brilliant – when shopping, just remember, generally you get what you pay for.

BIGGING UP FRESH HERBS

Herbs are a gift to any cook, and I use them loads in this book. Instead of buying them, why not grow them yourself in the garden or in a pot on your windowsill? Herbs are the foundation of all cooking, allowing you to add single-minded flavour to a dish, without the need to over-season, which is good for everyone. They're also packed with all sorts of incredible qualities on the nutritional front – we like that.

MIGHTY MEAT & EGGS

I've said it before and I stand by it – there's no point in eating meat unless the animal was raised well, free to roam, lived in an unstressful environment and it was at optimal health. It makes total sense to me that what we put into our bodies should have lived a good life, to in turn give us goodness. Generally speaking, we should all be striving to eat more plant-based meals that hero veg, beans and pulses, and enjoying better-quality meat, less often. With this in mind, please choose organic, free-range or higher-welfare meat whenever you can, making sure beef or lamb is grass fed. The same goes for eggs and anything containing egg, such as noodles and pasta – always choose free-range or organic. Please choose organic stock, too.

FOCUSING ON FISH

It's really important to buy fish at its freshest. It's obvious, but the minute you buy fish and take it out of the environment it's stored in, the quality starts to decrease. Buy fish at its best and use it on the same day. If you can't use it that day, freeze it until you need it, or even buy quality frozen, tinned or jarred fish, which can also be fantastic. Make sure you choose responsibly sourced wherever possible – look for the MSC logo, or talk to your fishmonger or the guys at the fish counter in your local supermarket and take their advice. Try to mix up your choices, choosing seasonal, sustainable options as they're available.

DIALLING UP YOUR DAIRY

With staple dairy products, like milk, yoghurt and butter, I couldn't endorse more the trade-up to organic. It is slightly more expensive, but we're talking about pennies not pounds, so this is a much easier trade-up than meat. Plus, every time you buy organic, you vote for a better food system.

LET'S CHAT EQUIPMENT

I've kept the equipment I've used in this book pretty simple – a set of saucepans and non-stick ovenproof frying pans, a griddle and a shallow casserole pan, chopping boards, some sturdy roasting trays and a decent set of knives (and a couple of baking tins if you're eyeing up the sweet chapter) will see you through. If you want to save time, there are a few kitchen gadgets that will make your life a lot easier – things like a speed-peeler, a box grater and a pestle and mortar are all fantastic for creating great texture and boosting flavour, and a food processor is always a bonus, especially if you're short on time! Keep your kit in good nick, and your kitchen organized, and you'll be ready to go.

SALADS

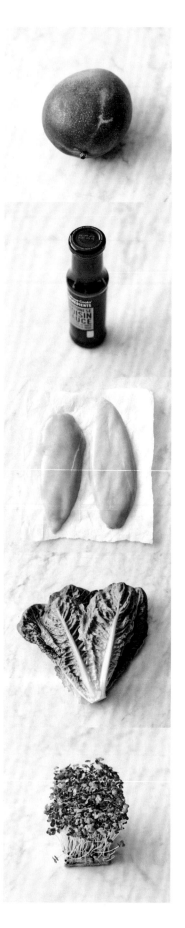

HOISIN CHICKEN LETTUCE CUPS

SERVES 2   TOTAL 17 MINUTES

1 ripe mango

2 tablespoons hoisin sauce

2 x 120g skinless chicken breasts

1 romaine lettuce (300g)

1 punnet of cress

Put a griddle pan on a high heat. Cut the two cheeks off the mango, slice each into three lengthways, then slice off the skin and discard. Dice all the flesh into 1 cm cubes. Scrunch the stone over a bowl, to extract any pulp and juice, mix with the hoisin to make a dressing, and divide between two little pots.

Flatten the chicken breasts by pounding them with your fists until the fat end is the same thickness as the skinny end. Rub with 1 tablespoon of olive oil and a pinch of sea salt and black pepper, then griddle for 2 to 3 minutes on each side, or until bar-marked and cooked through. Meanwhile, trim the lettuce, click the leaves apart and divide between two plates, snipping the cress alongside.

Divide up the mango and the hoisin pots. Slice the chicken and arrange on the plates, then tuck in, using the lettuce cups as a receptacle to hold everything.

CALORIES	FAT	SAT FAT	PROTEIN	CARBS	SUGAR	SALT	FIBRE
289kcal	9.6g	1.8g	31.3g	20.3g	19.2g	1.3g	2.5g

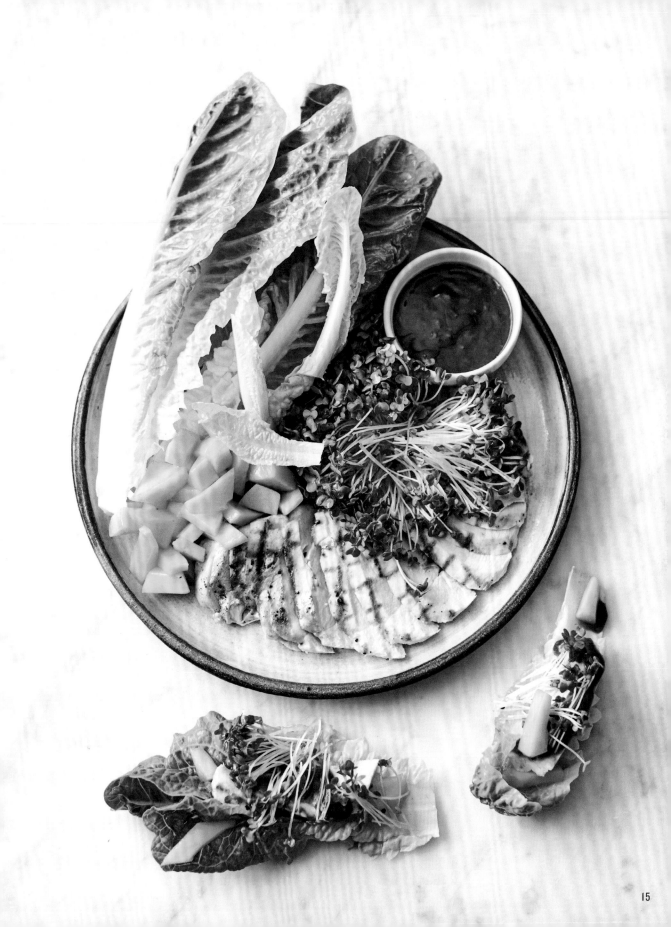

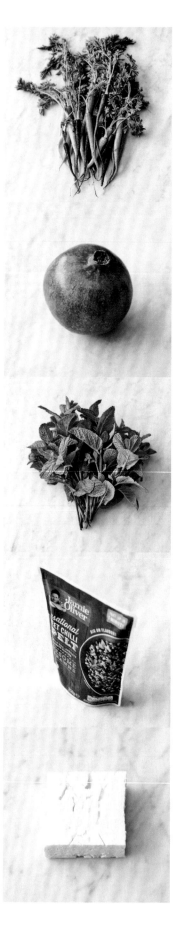

CARROT & GRAIN SALAD

SERVES 2   TOTAL 18 MINUTES

350g mixed-colour baby heritage carrots

1 pomegranate

1 big bunch of fresh mint (60g)

1 x 250g packet of mixed cooked grains

40g feta cheese

Wash the carrots, halve any larger ones, then place in a large cold non-stick frying pan with 1 tablespoon of olive oil and a pinch of sea salt and black pepper. Put on a medium-high heat for 15 minutes, or until golden and tender, tossing regularly. Meanwhile, halve the pomegranate, squeeze the juice from one half through a sieve into a large bowl, add 1 tablespoon of red wine vinegar and 2 teaspoons of extra virgin olive oil. Finely chop the top leafy half of the mint (reserving a few nice leaves), stir into the bowl, then taste and season to perfection.

Transfer the carrots to the dressing bowl, while you toss the grains in the pan for 1 minute with a splash of water to warm through. Tip into the bowl and mix with the dressed carrots, then divide between your plates.

Holding the remaining pomegranate half cut side down in your fingers, bash the back of it with a spoon so all the seeds tumble over the salads. Crumble or grate over the feta, sprinkle over the reserved mint leaves, and tuck in.

CALORIES	FAT	SAT FAT	PROTEIN	CARBS	SUGAR	SALT	FIBRE
477kcal	23.7g	5.7g	15.5g	49.1g	1.7g	1.2g	11.3g

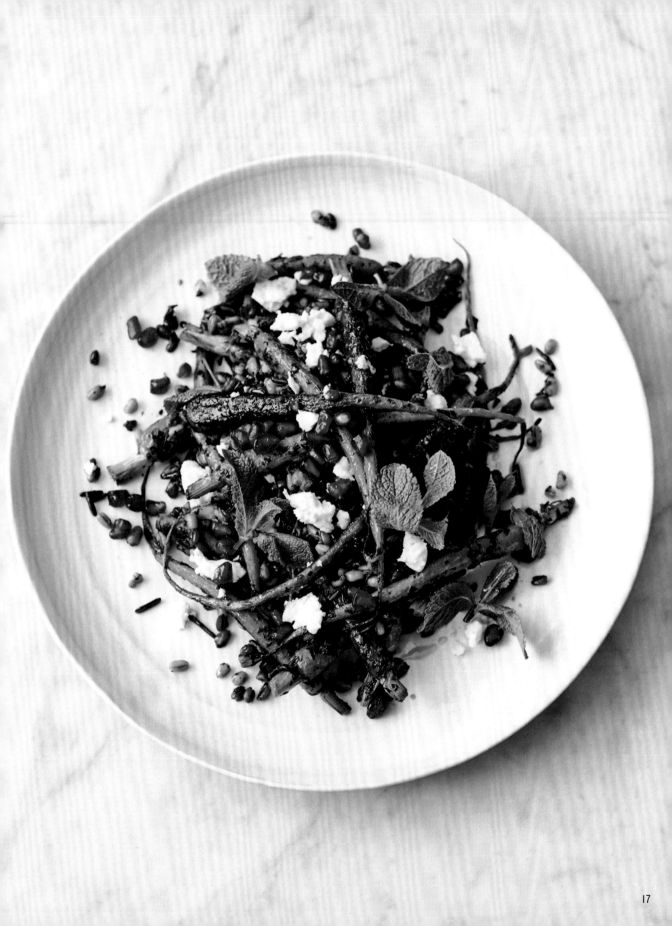

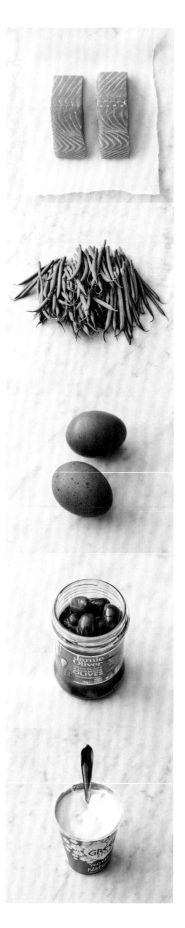

SORTA SALMON NIÇOISE

SERVES 2   TOTAL 18 MINUTES

2 x 120g salmon fillets, skin on, scaled, pin-boned

300g green beans

2 large eggs

8 black olives (stone in)

2 heaped tablespoons Greek yoghurt

Place the salmon skin side down in a colander over a pan of boiling salted water, covered, to steam for 8 minutes. Line up the beans, trim off just the stalk end, then boil in the water under the salmon for 6 minutes, or until just cooked but not squeaky. Gently lower in the eggs to cook for exactly 5½ minutes, alongside. Meanwhile, squash the olives and remove the stones, then finely chop the flesh. Mix half of the olives through the yoghurt with a splash of red wine vinegar, taste and season to perfection with sea salt and black pepper.

Remove the salmon to a board, then drain the eggs and beans in the colander. Toss the beans in the dressing and divide between your plates. Refresh the eggs under cold water until cool enough to handle, then peel and cut into quarters. Flake over the salmon, discarding the skin, arrange the eggs on top and dot over the remaining chopped olives. Finish with 1 teaspoon of extra virgin olive oil and a good pinch of pepper, from a height.

CALORIES	FAT	SAT FAT	PROTEIN	CARBS	SUGAR	SALT	FIBRE
398kcal	24.7g	6g	38.3g	6.5g	5.2g	0.7g	3.3g

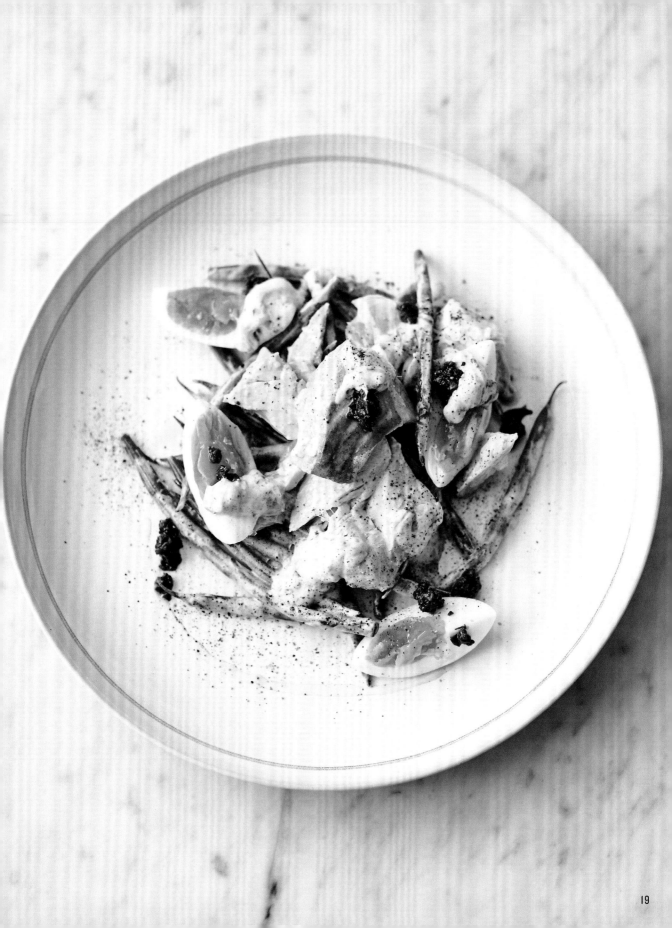

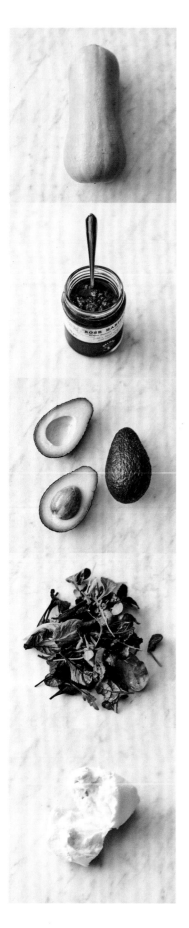

HARISSA SQUASH SALAD

SERVES 4 | FAST PREP 10 MINUTES | COOK 50 MINUTES

1 butternut squash (1.2kg)

1 heaped tablespoon rose harissa

2 ripe avocados

100g mixed salad leaves

1 x 125g ball of mozzarella cheese

Preheat the oven to 180°C/350°F/gas 4. Carefully cut the squash into rough 5cm chunks (seeds and all), then, in a roasting tray, rub all over with the harissa, 1 tablespoon of olive oil and a pinch of sea salt and black pepper. Roast for 50 minutes, or until soft, golden and gnarly.

With a few minutes to go, place 1 tablespoon each of extra virgin olive oil and red wine vinegar, and a little salt and pepper, in a large bowl. Halve, peel, destone, slice and toss in the avocados, then gently mix in the salad leaves. Use forks to divide and tear the hot squash (skin, seeds and all) between your plates. Divide up the salad on top and tear over the mozzarella, then serve.

CALORIES	FAT	SAT FAT	PROTEIN	CARBS	SUGAR	SALT	FIBRE
361kcal	24.2g	7.4g	11.1g	26.3g	14.2g	1.3g	5.6g

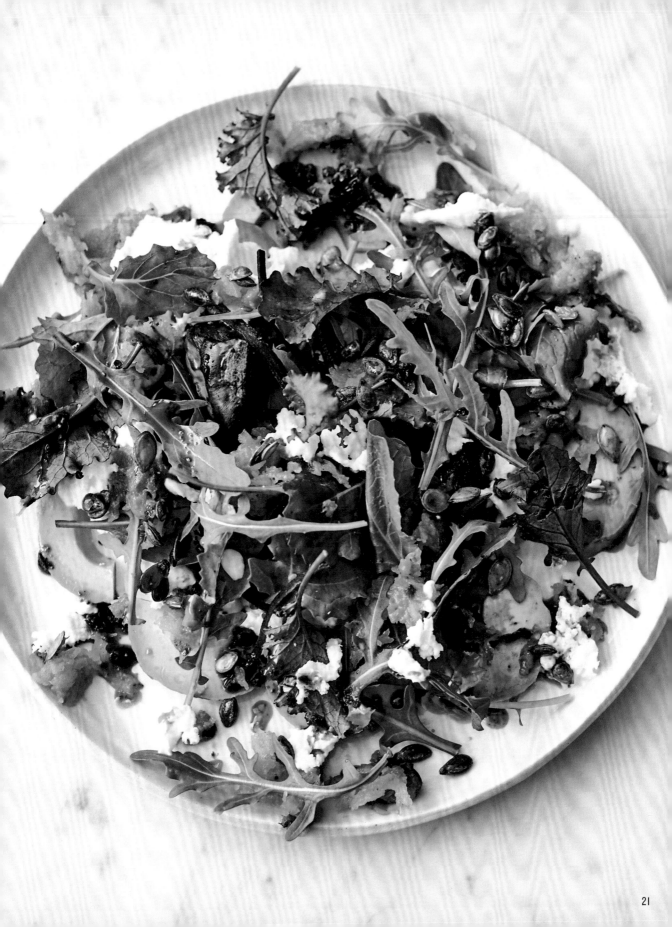

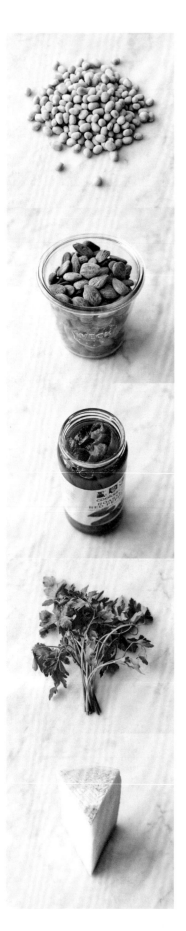

BROAD BEAN SALAD

SERVES 2   TOTAL JUST 15 MINUTES

200g fresh podded or frozen broad beans

30g whole almonds

1 x 480g jar of roasted red peppers in brine

½ a bunch of fresh flat-leaf parsley (15g)

30g Manchego cheese

Boil the beans in a pan of boiling salted water for 3 minutes, then drain and pinch the skins off any larger beans. Toast the almonds in a dry griddle pan on a medium heat until lightly golden, tossing regularly, then remove and finely slice.

Drain the peppers and open out flat, then char on the hot griddle until bar-marked on one side only. Remove and slice 1cm thick. Finely slice the parsley stalks, pick the leaves, then toss with the broad beans, peppers, 1½ tablespoons of extra virgin olive oil and 1 tablespoon each of red wine vinegar and brine from the pepper jar. Taste, season to perfection with sea salt and black pepper, and divide between your plates.

Finely shave over the cheese with a speed-peeler, drizzle with 1 teaspoon of extra virgin olive oil, scatter over the almonds, and serve.

CALORIES	FAT	SAT FAT	PROTEIN	CARBS	SUGAR	SALT	FIBRE
360kcal	26.7g	5.8g	14.3g	15.2g	8g	0.4g	8.2g

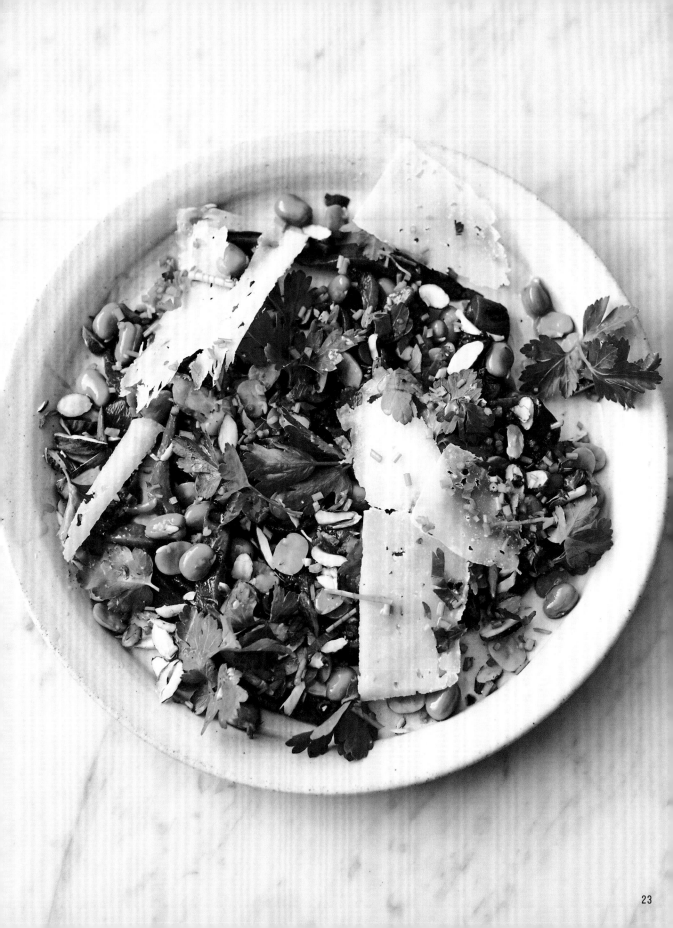

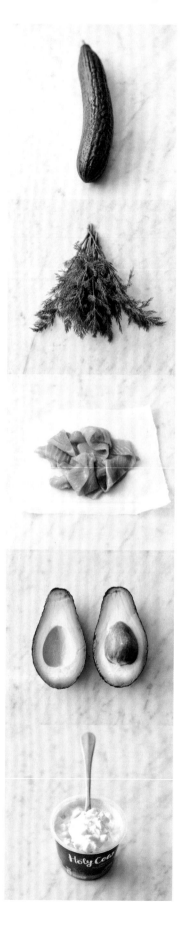

SMOKED SALMON PLATES

SERVES 2   TOTAL JUST 15 MINUTES

1 small cucumber

6 sprigs of fresh dill

100g smoked salmon

1 ripe avocado

2 tablespoons cottage cheese

Use a speed-peeler to strip the cucumber lengthways into fine ribbons. In a bowl, toss it with a small pinch of sea salt and 2 tablespoons of red wine vinegar, and scrunch to quickly pickle it. Pick and mix in most of the dill.

Drape and divide the smoked salmon between two plates. Halve, destone, peel and add the avocado. Pile the cucumber ribbons delicately to one side, filling the avocado halves with the cucumber liquor. Spoon over the cottage cheese, then drizzle with 1 teaspoon of extra virgin olive oil, add a pinch of black pepper from a height, pick over the remaining dill, and tuck on in.

CALORIES	FAT	SAT FAT	PROTEIN	CARBS	SUGAR	SALT	FIBRE
246kcal	17.7g	3.9g	17.1g	4.4g	3.2g	1.5g	1.2g

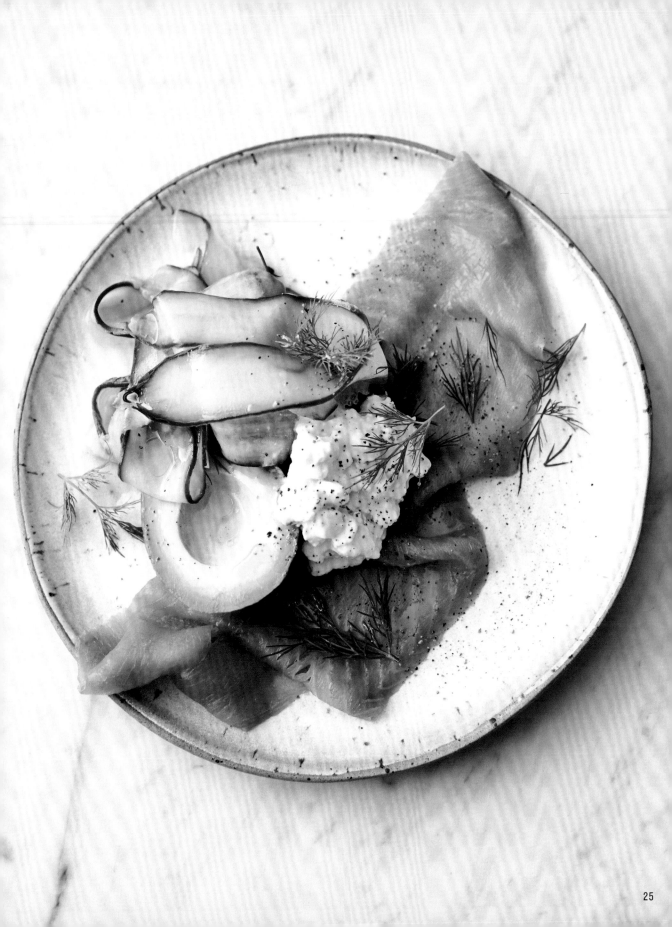

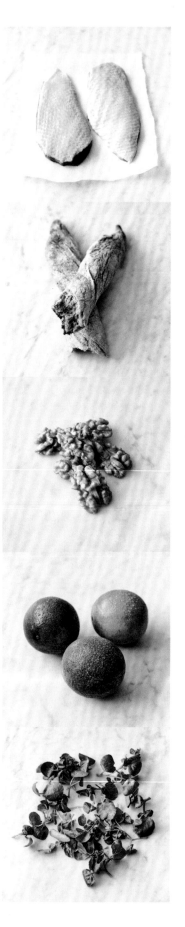

DUCK & ORANGE SALAD

SERVES 2   TOTAL 24 MINUTES

2 x 150g duck breast fillets, skin on

1 baguette

15g shelled unsalted walnut halves

3 regular or blood oranges

30g watercress

Score the duck skin, rub all over with sea salt and black pepper, then place skin side down in a large non-stick frying pan on a medium-high heat. Sear for 6 minutes, or until the skin is dark golden, then turn and cook for 5 minutes, or to your liking. Remove to a board to rest, leaving the pan on the heat.

Slice 10 thin slices of baguette (keeping the rest for another day). Place in the hot pan with the walnuts to toast and get golden in the duck fat, then remove and arrange the toasts on your plates. Meanwhile, top and tail the oranges, cut away the peel, then finely slice into rounds (removing any pips).

Finely slice the duck, place on the toasts, dotting any extra slices in between, then add the oranges in and around. Dress the watercress with any resting juices on the board, then sprinkle over. Finely grate or crumble over the walnuts, sprinkle from a height with a little extra seasoning, and serve.

CALORIES	FAT	SAT FAT	PROTEIN	CARBS	SUGAR	SALT	FIBRE
600kcal	20.5g	4.5g	49g	54.8g	26.9g	1.5g	6.1g

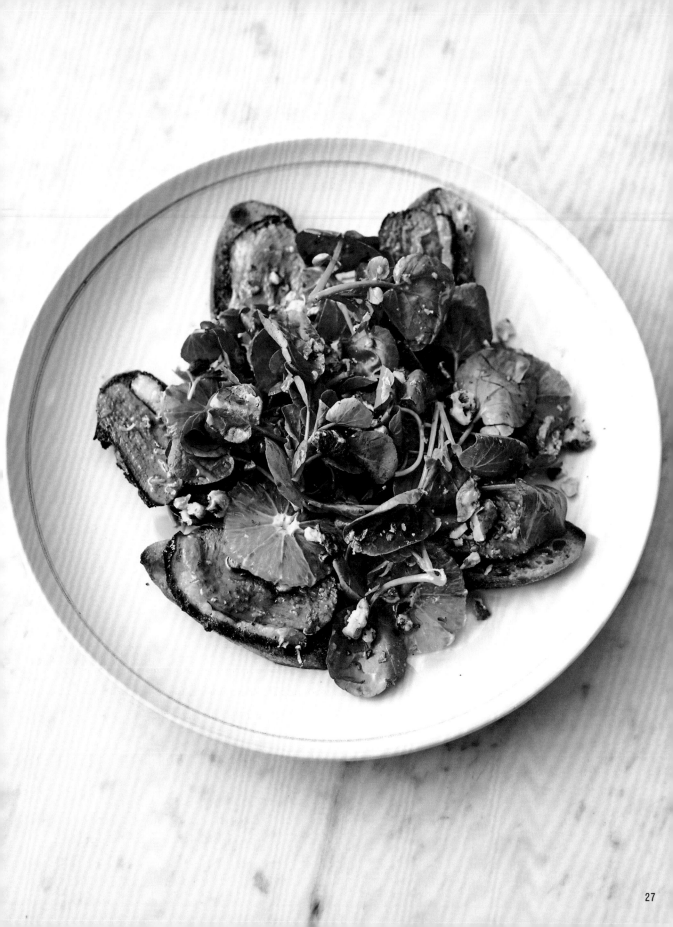

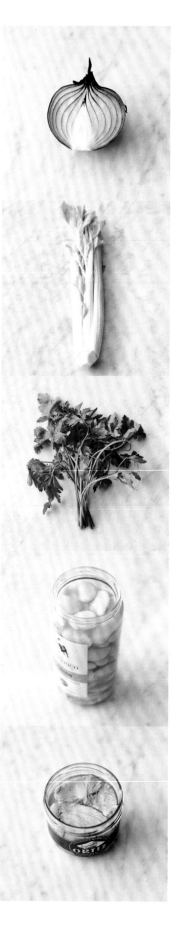

TUNA BUTTER BEAN SALAD

SERVES 2   TOTAL JUST 15 MINUTES

½ a red onion

1 celery heart

½ a bunch of fresh flat-leaf parsley (15g)

½ x 660g jar of butter beans

1 x 220g jar of tuna in olive oil

Peel the red onion and slice it as finely as you can. In a large bowl, scrunch it with ½ a tablespoon of red wine vinegar and a little pinch of sea salt. Trim and finely slice the celery and pile on top of the onion. Finely slice the parsley stalks, add to the bowl, then pick over the leaves.

Drain the beans and place in a single layer in a hot non-stick frying pan on a medium-high heat with 1 teaspoon of olive oil. Have faith, let them crisp up and get golden on the bottom, then turn so they crisp up on the other side.

Drizzle 1 tablespoon each of extra virgin olive oil and red wine vinegar over the onion salad, drain and flake in the tuna, then gently toss it all together. Divide the popped beans between your plates, pile the salad on top and sprinkle from a height with a good pinch of black pepper, then tuck in.

CALORIES	FAT	SAT FAT	PROTEIN	CARBS	SUGAR	SALT	FIBRE
362kcal	15.7g	2.2g	36.3g	19.3g	4.3g	1.5g	6.1g

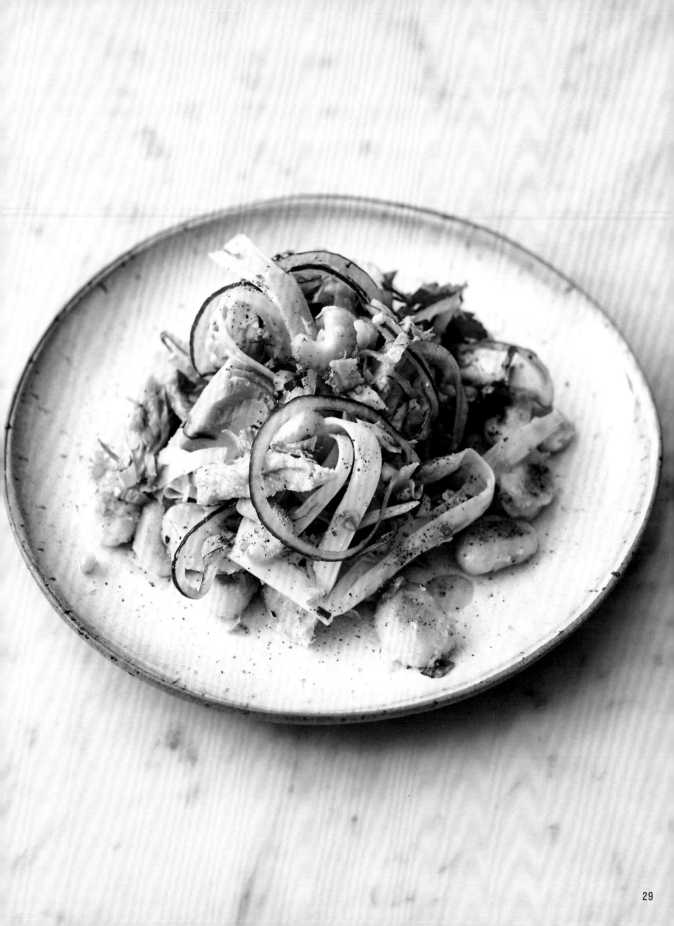

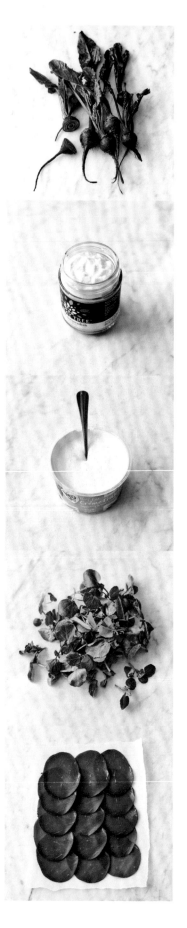

BEEF, BEETS & HORSERADISH

SERVES 2   TOTAL JUST 14 MINUTES

160g raw mixed-colour baby beets

3 heaped teaspoons creamed horseradish

3 heaped teaspoons half-fat crème fraîche

50g watercress

40g finely sliced bresaola

Scrub the beets clean, reserving any nice leaves, then finely slice into matchsticks with good knife skills or using the julienne cutter on a mandolin (use the guard!). Dress with ½ a tablespoon each of extra virgin olive oil and red wine vinegar, the horseradish and crème fraîche, then season to perfection with sea salt and black pepper. Delicately toss with the watercress and any reserved beet leaves.

Divide up the bresaola between your plates, followed by the beet salad, then drizzle with 1 teaspoon of extra virgin olive oil, and serve.

CALORIES	FAT	SAT FAT	PROTEIN	CARBS	SUGAR	SALT	FIBRE
154kcal	8.6g	2.9g	11.1g	8.5g	7.3g	0.8g	2.4g

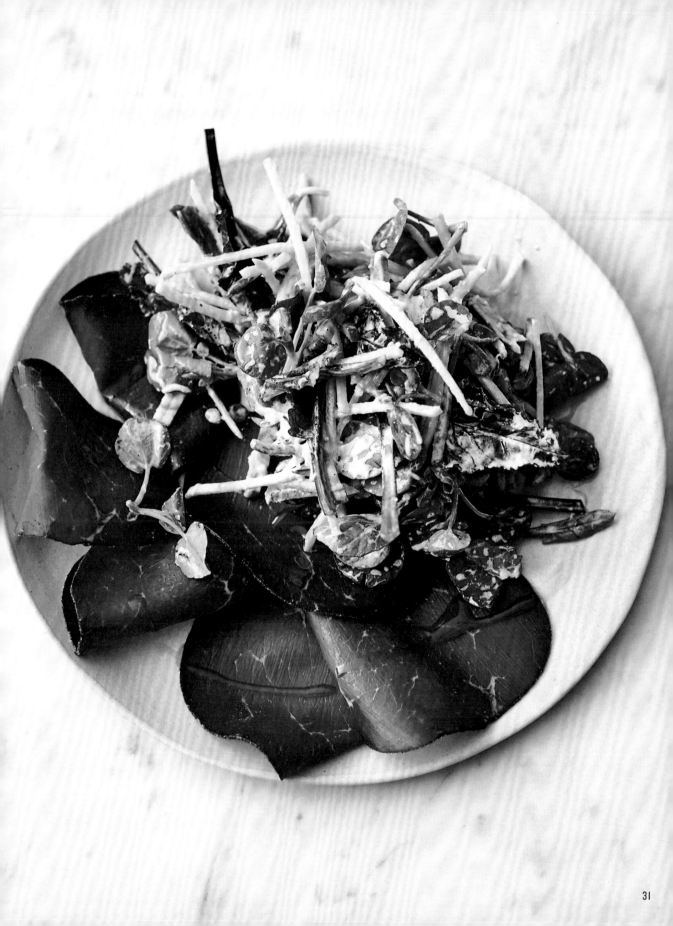

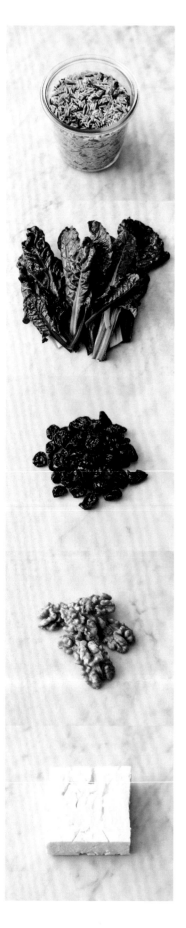

CHERRY CHARD WILD RICE

SERVES 2   TOTAL 28 MINUTES

150g mixed wild rice

200g mixed-colour chard

60g dried sour cherries

20g shelled unsalted walnut halves

40g feta cheese

Cook the rice in a pan of boiling salted water according to the packet instructions. Trim the chard stalks, cut them off and pop just the stalks into a colander, cover and steam above the rice for 3 minutes. Add the leaves and steam for another 2 minutes, then remove. Meanwhile, finely chop the cherries and, in a large bowl, mix with 1 tablespoon each of red wine vinegar and rice cooking water, then 1 tablespoon of extra virgin olive oil. Finely slice the walnuts, then the chard stalks, shred the leaves.

Drain the rice well, add to the cherry dressing bowl with all the chard and crumble in the feta. Toss well, then taste and season to perfection with sea salt and black pepper. Dish up, and sprinkle over the walnuts.

CALORIES	FAT	SAT FAT	PROTEIN	CARBS	SUGAR	SALT	FIBRE
548kcal	17.9g	4.6g	16g	84.3g	24.7g	1.1g	3.4g

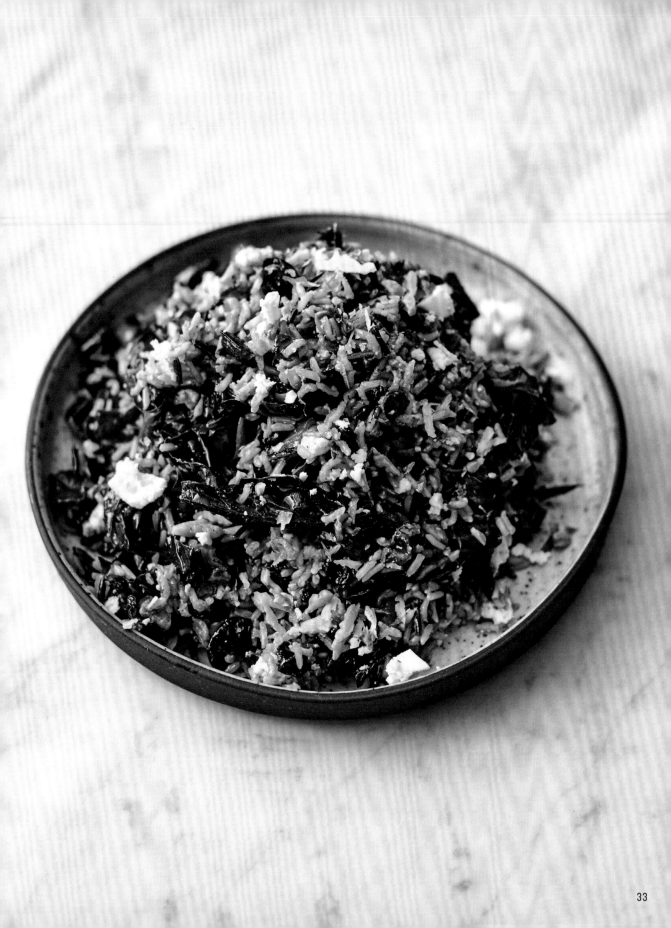

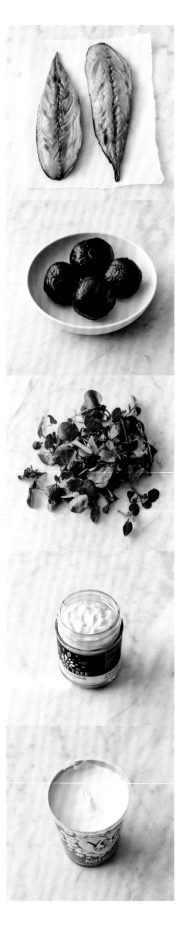

CRISPY SMOKED MACKEREL

SERVES 2 | TOTAL JUST 10 MINUTES

2 x 70g smoked mackerel fillets

300g vac-packed beetroots

50g watercress

2 teaspoons creamed horseradish (or use fresh, if you prefer)

2 tablespoons natural yoghurt

With a sharp knife, slash the mackerel skin at 1cm intervals, then place skin side down in a non-stick frying pan on a medium heat to get super golden and crisp. Meanwhile, drain the beets, saving the liquor. Finely slice the beets – I like to use a crinkle-cut knife. Arrange on your plates and pile the watercress on top.

Stir the horseradish into the yoghurt, then taste and season to perfection with sea salt and black pepper. Place the crispy mackerel on top of the salads, then dot around the horseradish yoghurt. Mix the beet juice with 1 tablespoon of extra virgin olive oil and drizzle over the top, then tuck in.

CALORIES	FAT	SAT FAT	PROTEIN	CARBS	SUGAR	SALT	FIBRE
352kcal	24.7g	5.1g	18g	14.2g	13.3g	1.5g	3.2g

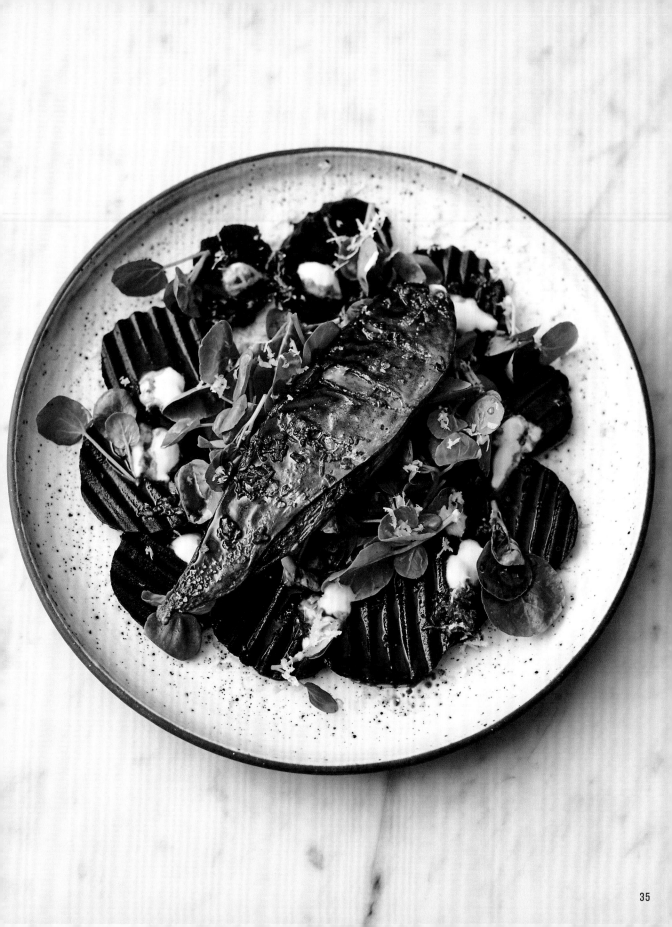

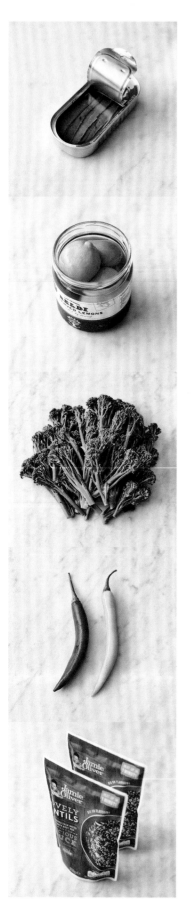

TASTY WARM LENTIL SALAD

SERVES 4   TOTAL JUST 13 MINUTES

1 x 50g tin of anchovies in oil

1 preserved lemon (20g)

400g tenderstem broccoli

1–2 fresh mixed-colour chillies

2 x 250g packets of cooked lentils

Put all the anchovies and their oil into a blender with 1 tablespoon of liquor from the preserved lemon jar and a splash of water. Blitz until smooth, loosening with a little more water, if needed.

Trim the broccoli and blanch in a large pan of boiling salted water for 3 minutes, or until just tender, while you quarter the preserved lemon and trim away the seedy core, then finely chop the rind. Finely slice the chillies. Drain the broccoli, return to the pan over the heat and toss with the lemon, most of the chilli and 1 tablespoon of extra virgin olive oil. Add the lentils and toss for 2 minutes, then divide between plates, drizzle over the anchovy dressing and scatter with the reserved chilli. Finish with ½ a tablespoon of extra virgin olive oil.

CALORIES	FAT	SAT FAT	PROTEIN	CARBS	SUGAR	SALT	FIBRE
200kcal	7.6g	1.5g	13.6g	19.6g	3.6g	1.3g	10.8g

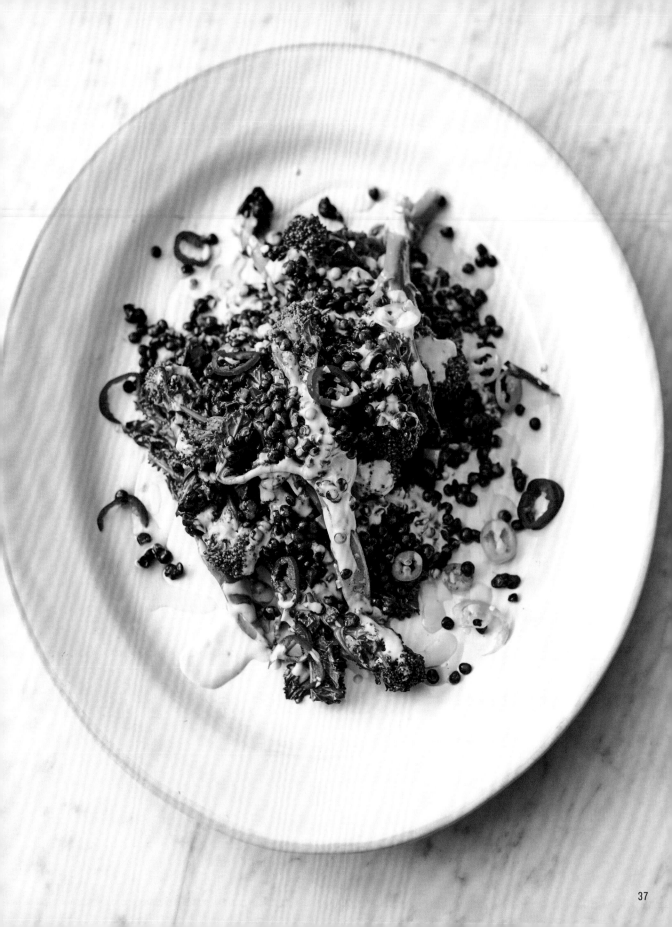

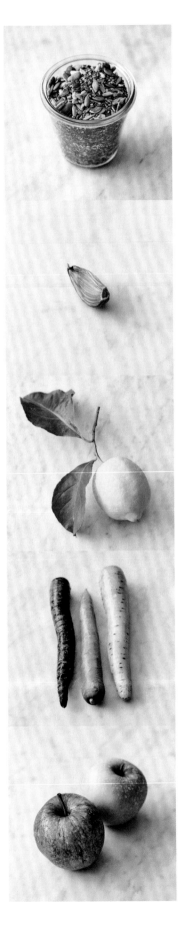

TAHINI CARROT SLAW

SERVES 2—4   TOTAL 20 MINUTES

2 heaped tablespoons mixed seeds

½ a clove of garlic

1 lemon

300g mixed-colour carrots

2 crunchy eating apples

Toast the seeds in a dry non-stick frying pan on a medium heat until lightly golden, tossing regularly, then remove. Put three-quarters of the seeds into a pestle and mortar with a pinch of sea salt, and pound until fairly fine. Peel and add the garlic, then smash to a paste. Squeeze in the lemon juice, then muddle in 1 tablespoon of extra virgin olive oil and a tiny dribble of red wine vinegar to make a delicious tahini-style dressing.

Wash the carrots, then finely slice into matchsticks with good knife skills or using the julienne cutter on a mandolin (use the guard!). Core and slice the apples the same way, then toss both with the tahini dressing. Taste, season to perfection with salt and black pepper, then scatter over the remaining seeds.

CALORIES	FAT	SAT FAT	PROTEIN	CARBS	SUGAR	SALT	FIBRE
263kcal	15.6g	2.4g	4.5g	27.9g	25.4g	0.6g	8g

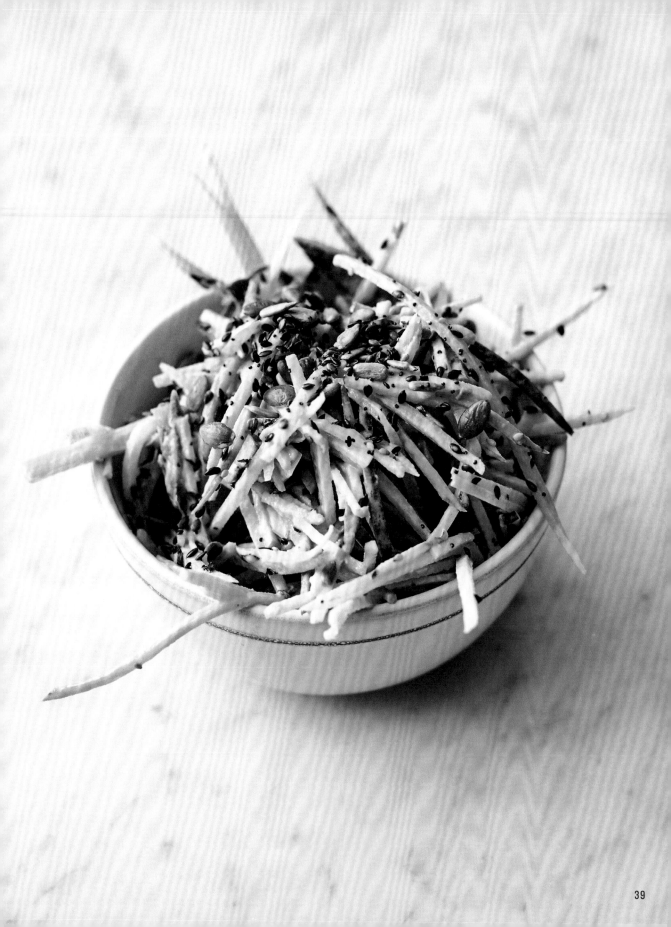

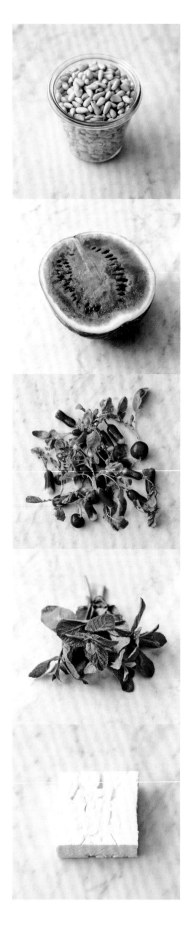

WATERMELON, RADISH & FETA SALAD

SERVES 2   TOTAL 18 MINUTES

2 tablespoons pine nuts

400g watermelon

200g radishes, ideally with leaves

4 sprigs of fresh mint

50g feta cheese

Toast the pine nuts in a dry non-stick frying pan on a medium heat for 1 minute, or until lightly golden, tossing regularly, then remove. Cut off the watermelon rind, pick out any seeds, then slice as finely as you can. Very finely slice the radishes, keeping any nice leaves attached, then gently dress both with 1 tablespoon of extra virgin olive oil and 2 tablespoons of red wine vinegar. Taste and season to perfection with sea salt and black pepper.

Arrange the watermelon and radishes on your plates or a sharing platter, sprinkle over the pine nuts, then pick over the mint leaves. Crumble over the feta, and finish with a pinch of pepper from a height.

CALORIES	FAT	SAT FAT	PROTEIN	CARBS	SUGAR	SALT	FIBRE
262kcal	18.7g	5g	7.1g	17g	16.9g	0.7g	0g

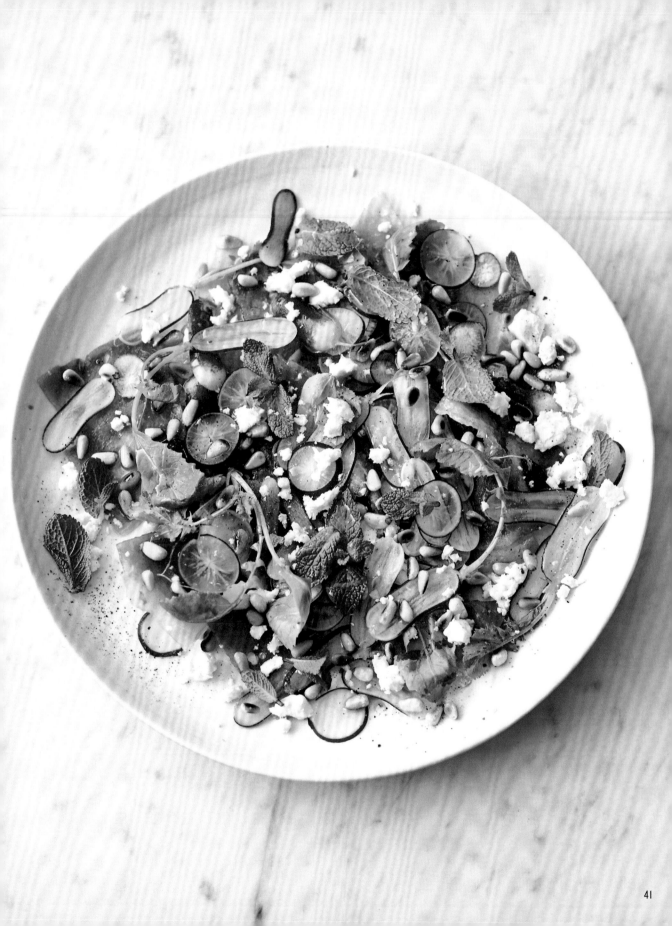

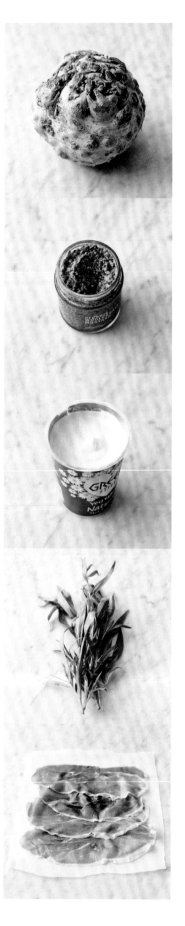

PROSCIUTTO CELERIAC SALAD

SERVES 2   TOTAL JUST 10 MINUTES

200g celeriac

2 teaspoons wholegrain mustard

2 heaped tablespoons Greek yoghurt

½ a bunch of fresh tarragon (15g)

4 slices of prosciutto

Peel the celeriac, then finely slice into matchsticks with good knife skills, using the julienne cutter on a mandolin (use the guard!), or a coarse box grater.

In a bowl, dress the celeriac with the mustard, yoghurt and 1 tablespoon each of extra virgin olive oil and red wine vinegar. Scrunch and massage together. Pick in the tarragon leaves, mix well, then taste and season to perfection with sea salt and black pepper. Divide between two plates, then wrap the prosciutto in waves around the outside. Drizzle with 1 teaspoon of extra virgin olive oil and sprinkle from a height with a pinch of pepper.

CALORIES	FAT	SAT FAT	PROTEIN	CARBS	SUGAR	SALT	FIBRE
192kcal	14.4g	3.7g	10.9g	4.8g	3.8g	1.5g	3.7g

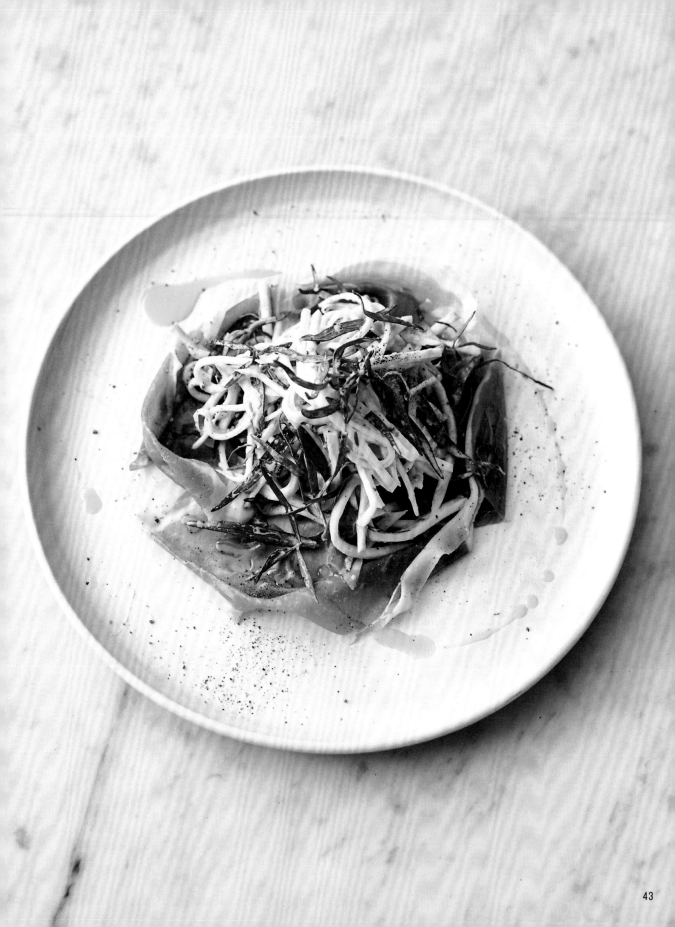

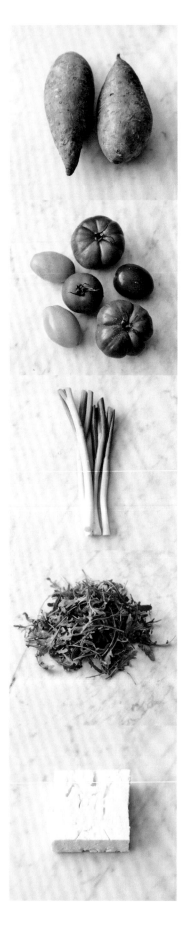

SWEET POTATO SALAD

SERVES 2   FAST PREP 9 MINUTES   SLOW COOK 1 HOUR

2 large sweet potatoes (300g each)

500g ripe mixed-colour tomatoes

4 spring onions

50g rocket

40g feta cheese

Preheat the oven to 180°C/350°F/gas 4. Scrub the sweet potatoes clean, place in a roasting tray and bake for 1 hour, or until soft through.

Once done, roughly chop the tomatoes, trim and finely slice the spring onions, then toss it all with 1 tablespoon of extra virgin olive oil and a splash of red wine vinegar. Taste and season to perfection with sea salt and black pepper.

Tear the soft sweet potatoes between two plates. Toss the rocket through the tomatoes, then pile on top. Crumble over the feta, drizzle with 1 teaspoon of extra virgin olive oil and sprinkle from a height with a pinch of pepper.

CALORIES	FAT	SAT FAT	PROTEIN	CARBS	SUGAR	SALT	FIBRE
429kcal	13.2g	4.4g	9.8g	72.5g	25.7g	1.1g	3.2g

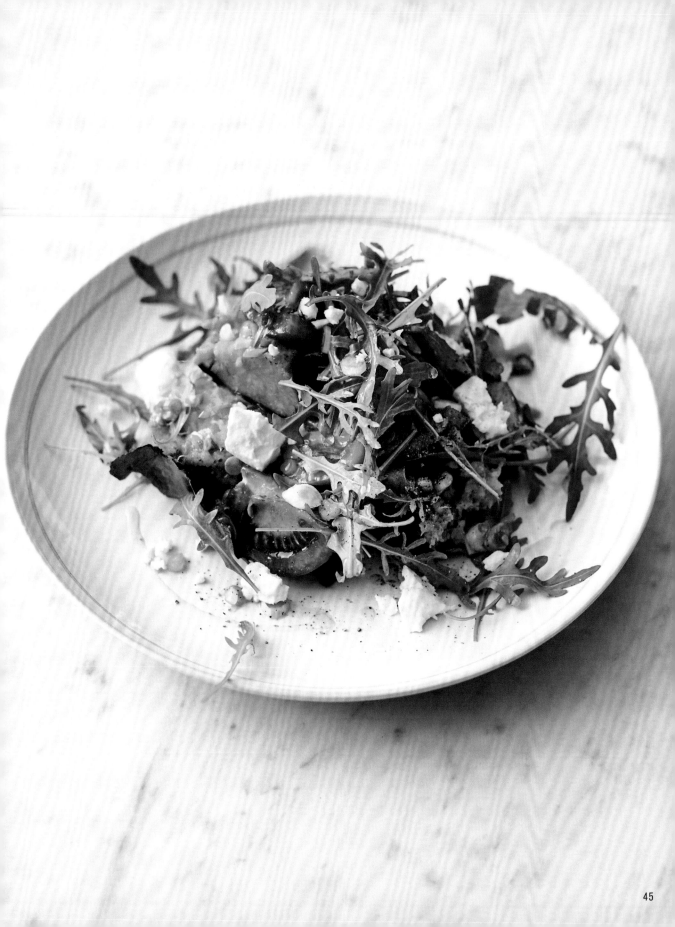

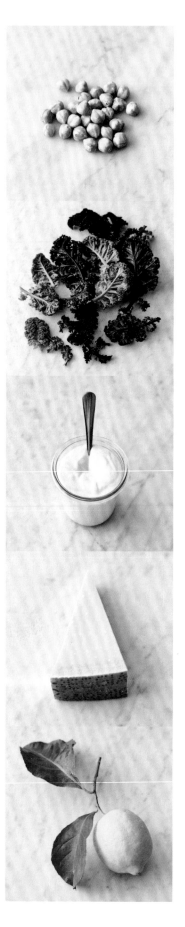

NUTTY KALE SALAD

SERVES 2 | TOTAL JUST 14 MINUTES

20g blanched hazelnuts

200g mixed-colour kale

60ml buttermilk

30g Parmesan cheese

1 lemon

Toast the hazelnuts in a dry non-stick frying pan on a medium heat until lightly golden, tossing often, then remove and randomly crush and finely slice them.

Tear off and discard any tough kale stalks, then roll up the leaves and slice super-finely, putting them into a large bowl as you go. Drizzle with 2 tablespoons of extra virgin olive oil, then add the buttermilk and half the nuts. Finely grate in half the Parmesan and all the lemon zest, then squeeze in half the juice. Scrunch and massage the kale to soften it. Taste and season to perfection with sea salt and black pepper, adding extra lemon juice, if you like.

Plate up, finely grate over the remaining Parmesan and scatter over the rest of the hazelnuts, then drizzle with 1 teaspoon of extra virgin olive oil.

CALORIES	FAT	SAT FAT	PROTEIN	CARBS	SUGAR	SALT	FIBRE
292kcal	25.8g	3.5g	11.3g	3.9g	3.6g	0.4g	0.7g

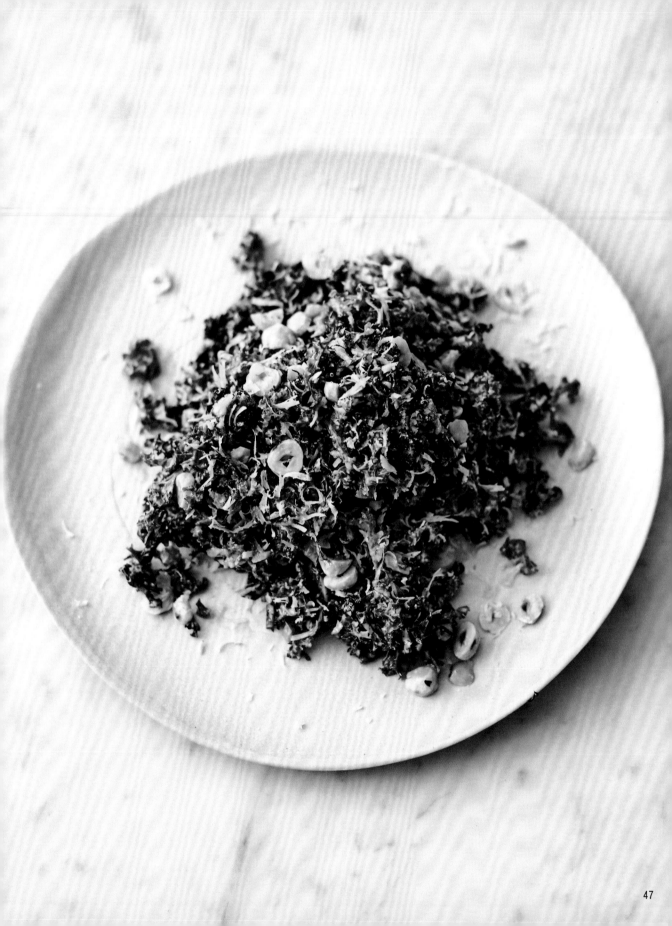

PASTA

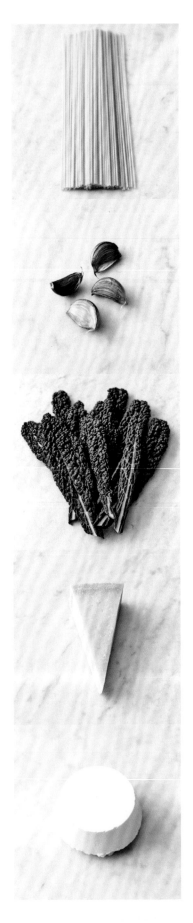

SUPER GREEN SPAGHETTI

SERVES 2   TOTAL JUST 13 MINUTES

150g dried spaghetti

4 cloves of garlic

200g cavolo nero

30g Parmesan cheese

30g ricotta cheese

Cook the pasta in a pan of boiling salted water according to the packet instructions. Meanwhile, peel the garlic. Tear the stems out of the cavolo and discard, adding the leaves and the garlic to the pasta pan for 5 minutes. Pour 1½ tablespoons of extra virgin olive oil into a blender, then finely grate in the Parmesan. Use tongs to carefully transfer the cavolo leaves and garlic straight into the blender and blitz for a few minutes until super-smooth. Taste and season to perfection with sea salt and black pepper.

Drain the pasta, reserving a mugful of cooking water. Return it to the pan and toss with the vibrant green sauce, loosening with a splash of reserved cooking water, if needed, then divide between your plates. Dot over the ricotta, drizzle with a tiny bit of extra virgin olive oil, and tuck right in.

CALORIES	FAT	SAT FAT	PROTEIN	CARBS	SUGAR	SALT	FIBRE
456kcal	17.3g	5.5g	18.4g	60.5g	3.7g	0.9g	2.6g

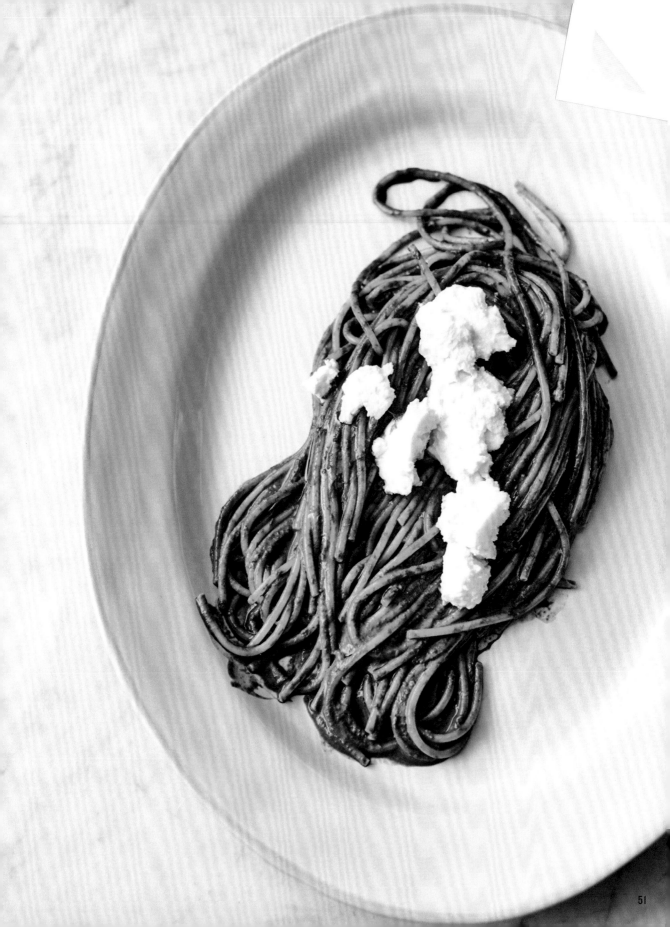

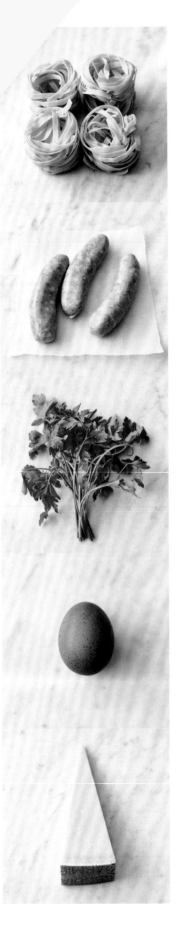

EASY SAUSAGE CARBONARA

SERVES 2 | TOTAL JUST 15 MINUTES

150g dried tagliatelle

3 sausages

½ a bunch of fresh flat-leaf parsley (15g)

1 large egg

30g Parmesan cheese

Cook the pasta in a pan of boiling salted water according to the packet instructions, then drain, reserving a mugful of cooking water. Meanwhile, squeeze the sausagemeat out of the skins, then, with wet hands, quickly shape into 18 even-sized balls. Roll and coat them in black pepper, then cook in a non-stick frying pan on a medium heat with ½ a tablespoon of olive oil until golden and cooked through, tossing regularly, then turn the heat off.

Finely chop the parsley, stalks and all, beat it with the egg and a splash of pasta cooking water, then finely grate and mix in most of the Parmesan.

Toss the drained pasta into the sausage pan, pour in the egg mixture, and toss for 1 minute off the heat (the egg will gently cook in the residual heat). Loosen with a good splash of reserved cooking water, season to perfection with sea salt and pepper, and finely grate over the remaining Parmesan.

CALORIES	FAT	SAT FAT	PROTEIN	CARBS	SUGAR	SALT	FIBRE
633kcal	30.6g	10.8g	33.6g	59.3g	3.1g	1.7g	2.6g

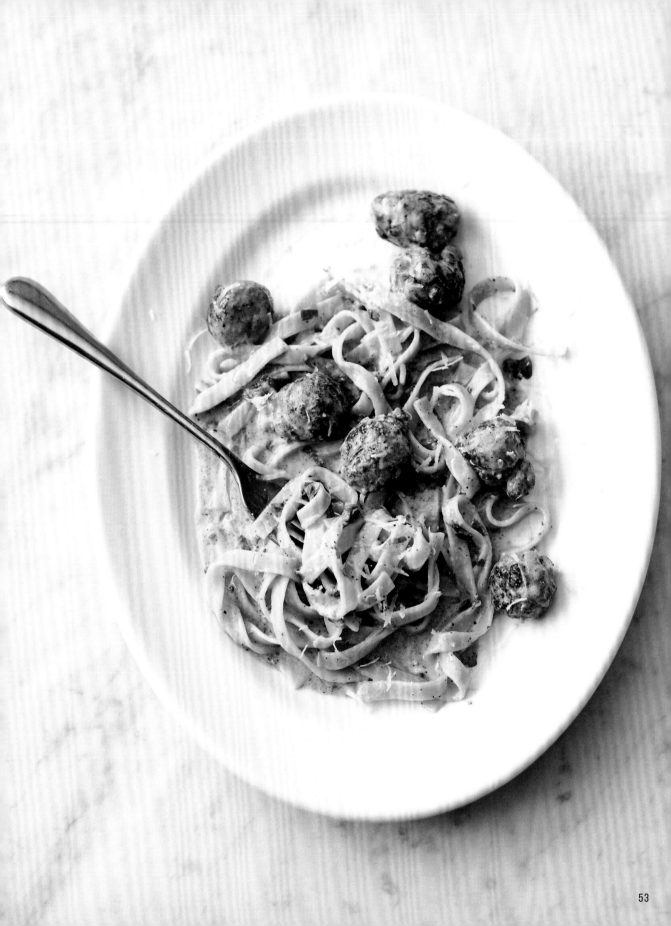

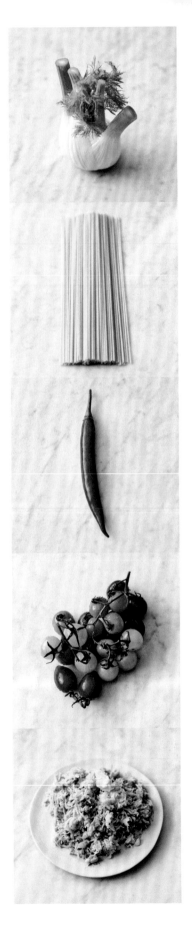

CRAB & FENNEL SPAGHETTI

SERVES 2   TOTAL 18 MINUTES

1 bulb of fennel

150g dried spaghetti

1 fresh red chilli

160g ripe mixed-colour cherry tomatoes

160g mixed brown & white crabmeat

Put a large non-stick frying pan on a medium-low heat. Trim the fennel, pick and reserve any leafy tops, then halve the bulb and finely slice it. Place in the pan with 1 tablespoon of olive oil and cook with the lid on for 5 minutes. Meanwhile, cook the pasta in a pan of boiling salted water according to the packet instructions, then drain, reserving a mugful of cooking water.

Deseed and finely slice the chilli, stir into the fennel pan and cook uncovered until soft and sticky, stirring occasionally. Halve the tomatoes and toss into the pan for 2 minutes, followed by the crabmeat and, 1 minute later, the drained pasta. Loosen with a splash of reserved cooking water, if needed, then season to perfection with sea salt and black pepper, sprinkle over any reserved fennel tops and drizzle with 1 teaspoon of extra virgin olive oil. Enjoy.

CALORIES	FAT	SAT FAT	PROTEIN	CARBS	SUGAR	SALT	FIBRE
464kcal	13.2g	2.6g	26.1g	63.9g	8.6g	1.1g	3.5g

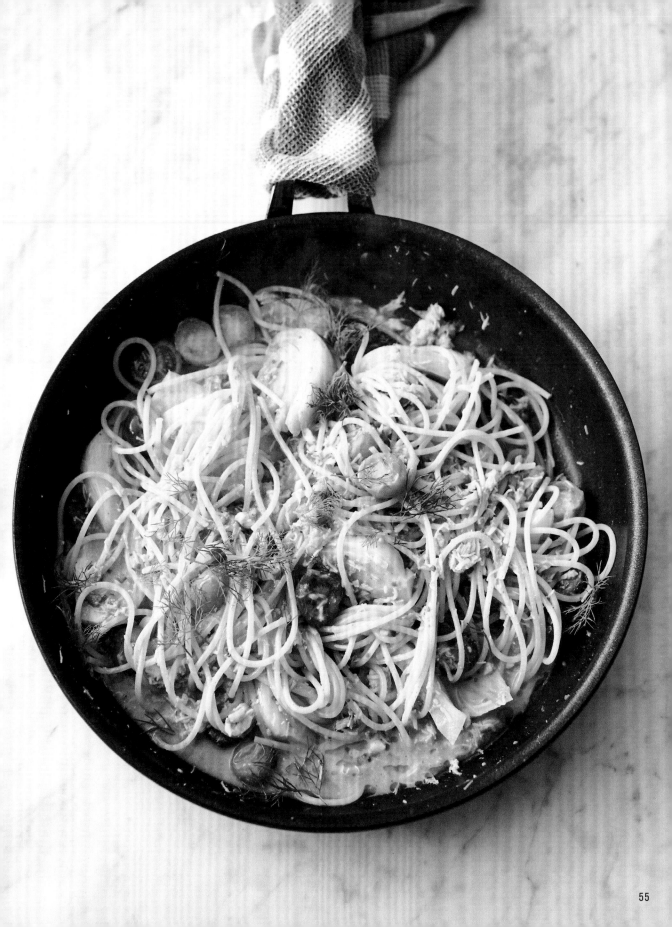

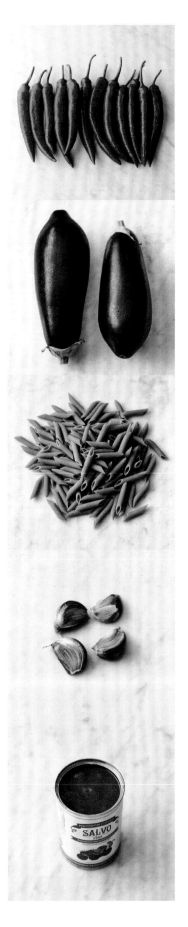

AUBERGINE PENNE ARRABBIATA

SERVES 4   TOTAL 28 MINUTES

12 fresh mixed-colour chillies

2 aubergines (500g total)

300g dried wholewheat penne

4 cloves of garlic

1 x 400g tin of plum tomatoes

To make a quick chilli oil, halve and deseed the chillies. Fill a clean heatproof jar with olive oil, then pour it into a non-stick frying pan on a medium-low heat and add the chillies to confit. Meanwhile, put a pan of boiling salted water on for the pasta. Halve the aubergines lengthways and blanch in the water, covered, for 5 minutes, then lift out, leaving the water on the boil. Carefully scoop the soft chillies into the jar, then spoon in the oil, leaving 2 tablespoons in the pan (keep the jar of chilli oil to add a kick to future meals). Chop the aubergine into 3cm chunks, add to the pan with a pinch of sea salt and black pepper, then turn the heat up to high, stirring regularly.

Cook the pasta according to the packet instructions while you peel and finely slice the garlic, then fry with the aubergine for 2 minutes. Pour in the tomatoes, breaking them up with a wooden spoon, and half a tin's worth of water. Add as many of the chillies as you dare to the sauce and simmer until the pasta is ready, then taste and season to perfection. Drain the pasta, reserving a mugful of cooking water, then toss the pasta through the sauce, loosening with a little reserved cooking water, if needed. Dish up.

CALORIES	FAT	SAT FAT	PROTEIN	CARBS	SUGAR	SALT	FIBRE
346kcal	9g	1.4g	12.8g	57.3g	9.5g	0.3g	7.1g

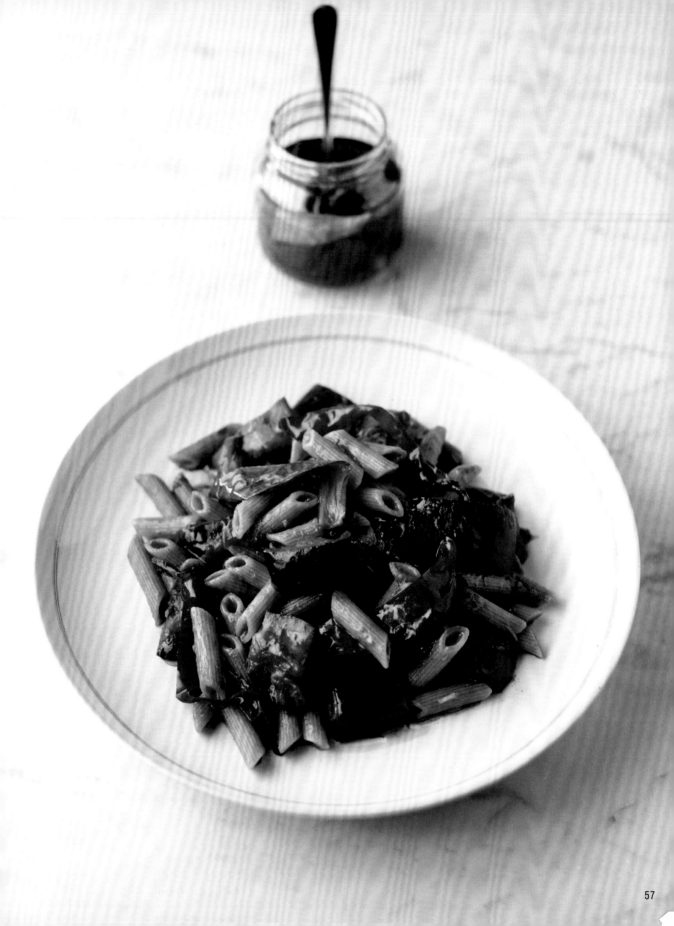

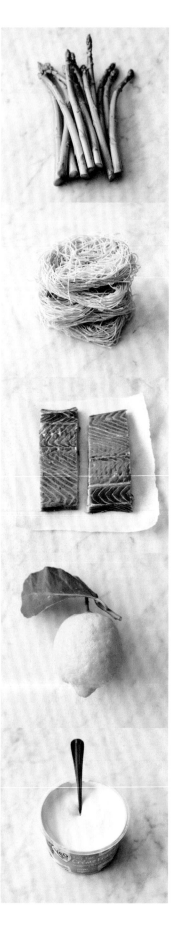

HOT-SMOKED SALMON PASTA

SERVES 4 | TOTAL JUST 12 MINUTES

350g asparagus

300g dried taglierini or angel-hair pasta

250g hot-smoked salmon, skin off

1 lemon

100ml half-fat crème fraîche

Use a speed-peeler to strip the top tender half of the asparagus stalks into ribbons. Finely slice the remaining stalks, discarding the woody ends. Cook the pasta in a pan of boiling salted water according to the packet instructions, then drain, reserving a mugful of cooking water. Meanwhile, roughly break the salmon into a large non-stick frying pan on a medium-high heat. Add the sliced asparagus stalks, and toss occasionally until the pasta's ready.

Finely grate half the lemon zest into the salmon pan, squeeze in half the juice, then toss in the drained pasta, a good splash of reserved cooking water and the crème fraîche. Add the asparagus ribbons, toss again, then season to perfection with sea salt and black pepper. Serve with lemon wedges, for squeezing over.

CALORIES	FAT	SAT FAT	PROTEIN	CARBS	SUGAR	SALT	FIBRE
435kcal	11.1g	4g	28.1g	59.3g	5.8g	1.4g	2.2g

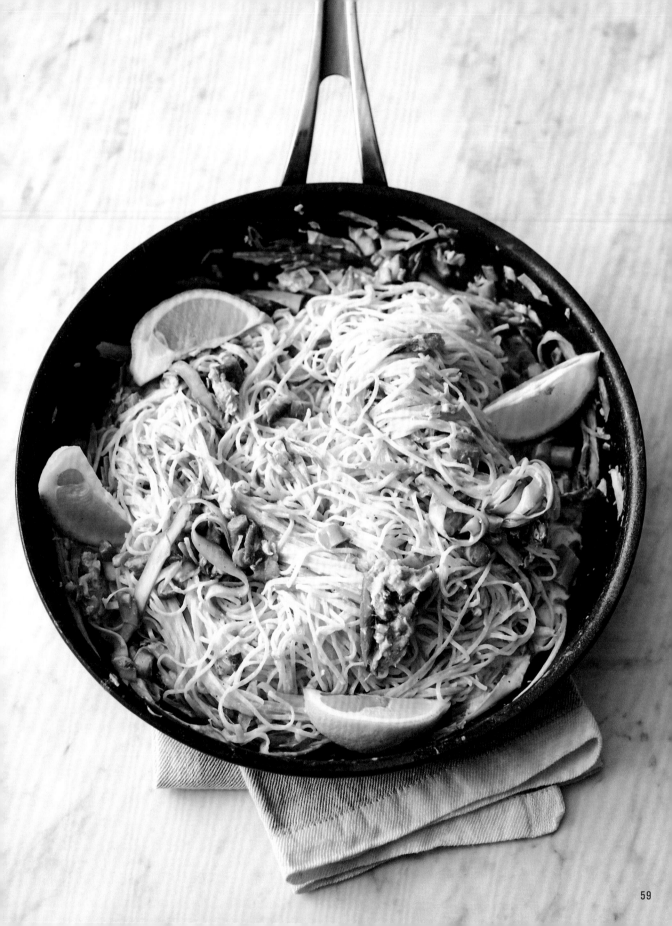

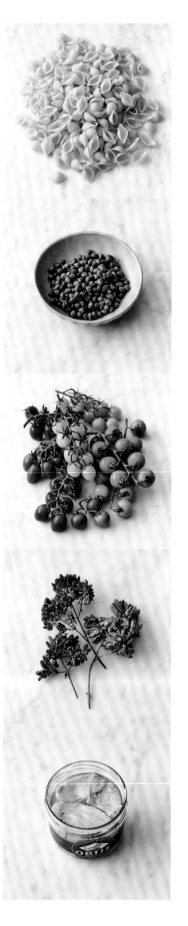

SICILIAN TUNA PASTA

SERVES 4   TOTAL JUST 14 MINUTES

300g dried pasta shells

4 heaped teaspoons baby capers

500g ripe mixed-colour cherry tomatoes

1 tablespoon dried oregano, ideally the flowering kind

1 x 220g jar of tuna in olive oil

Cook the pasta in a pan of boiling salted water according to the packet instructions. Meanwhile, place a large non-stick frying pan on a medium-high heat with 1 tablespoon of olive oil. Add the capers, fry until super-crispy, then scoop out and put aside, leaving the fragrant oil behind. Halve and add the tomatoes, then sprinkle in most of the oregano. Drain and flake in the tuna, add 2 ladlefuls of pasta cooking water, and simmer until the pasta is done.

Drain the pasta, reserving a mugful of cooking water, then toss the pasta into the tuna pan, loosening with a splash of reserved cooking water, if needed. Taste, season to perfection with sea salt and black pepper, then dish up. Sprinkle over the crispy capers and the remaining oregano from a height, drizzle with 1 teaspoon of extra virgin olive oil, and tuck in.

CALORIES	FAT	SAT FAT	PROTEIN	CARBS	SUGAR	SALT	FIBRE
411kcal	9.6g	1.3g	24.3g	60.7g	6.2g	1.1g	3.4g

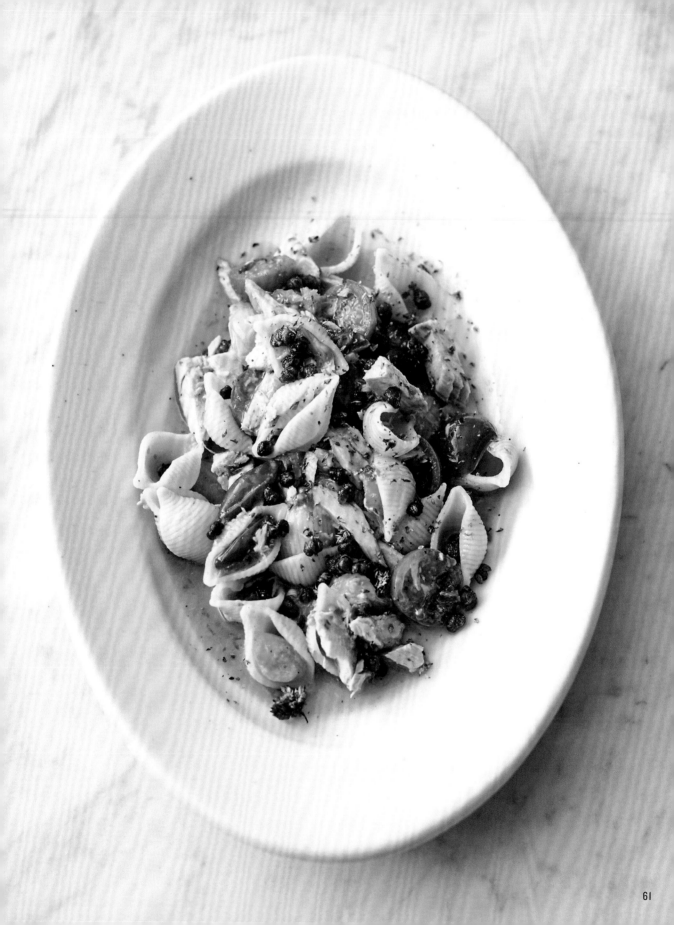

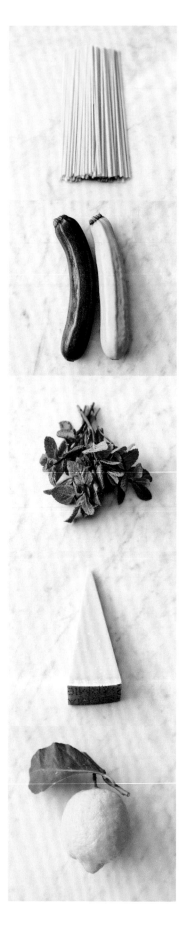

LEMONY COURGETTE LINGUINE

SERVES 2 | TOTAL JUST 15 MINUTES

150g dried linguine

2 mixed-colour courgettes

½ a bunch of fresh mint (15g)

30g Parmesan cheese

1 lemon

Cook the pasta in a pan of boiling salted water according to the packet instructions, then drain, reserving a mugful of cooking water. Meanwhile, slice the courgettes lengthways, then again into long matchsticks with good knife skills or using the julienne cutter on a mandolin (use the guard!). Place a large non-stick frying pan on a medium-high heat with 1 tablespoon of olive oil, then add the courgettes. Cook for 4 minutes, tossing regularly, while you finely slice the mint leaves, then stir them into the pan.

Toss the drained pasta into the courgette pan with a splash of reserved cooking water. Finely grate in most of the Parmesan and a little lemon zest, squeeze in all the juice, toss well, then taste and season to perfection with sea salt and black pepper. Dish up, finely grate over the remaining Parmesan and drizzle with 1 teaspoon of extra virgin olive oil before tucking in.

CALORIES	FAT	SAT FAT	PROTEIN	CARBS	SUGAR	SALT	FIBRE
430kcal	14.5g	4.4g	18.4g	60g	6.3g	0.8g	2.2g

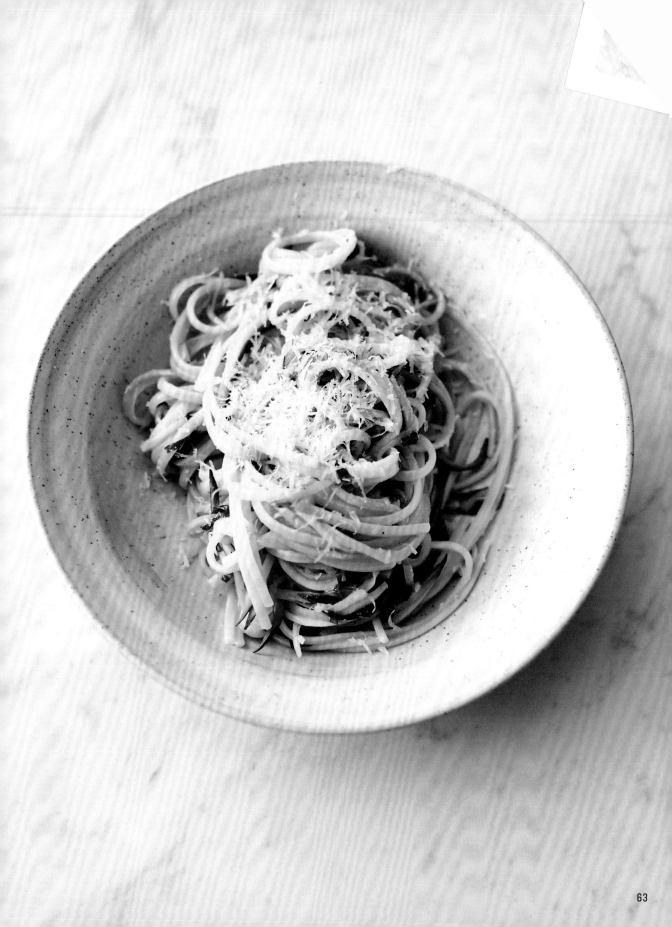

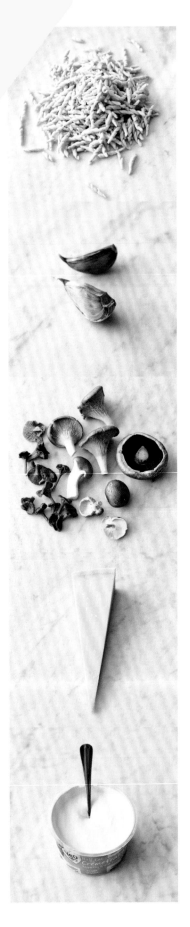

GARLIC MUSHROOM PASTA

SERVES 2　｜　TOTAL 16 MINUTES

150g dried trofie or fusilli

2 cloves of garlic

250g mixed mushrooms

25g Parmesan cheese

2 heaped tablespoons half-fat crème fraîche

Cook the pasta in a pan of boiling salted water according to the packet instructions, then drain, reserving a mugful of cooking water. Meanwhile, peel and finely slice the garlic. Place it in a large non-stick frying pan on a medium-high heat with ½ a tablespoon of olive oil, followed 1 minute later by the mushrooms, tearing up any larger ones. Season with sea salt and black pepper, and cook for 8 minutes, or until golden, tossing regularly.

Toss the drained pasta into the mushroom pan with a splash of reserved cooking water. Finely grate in most of the Parmesan, stir in the crème fraîche, taste, season to perfection, and dish up, finishing with a final grating of Parmesan.

CALORIES	FAT	SAT FAT	PROTEIN	CARBS	SUGAR	SALT	FIBRE
402kcal	13g	5.7g	16.8g	58.1g	3.7g	0.8g	3.6g

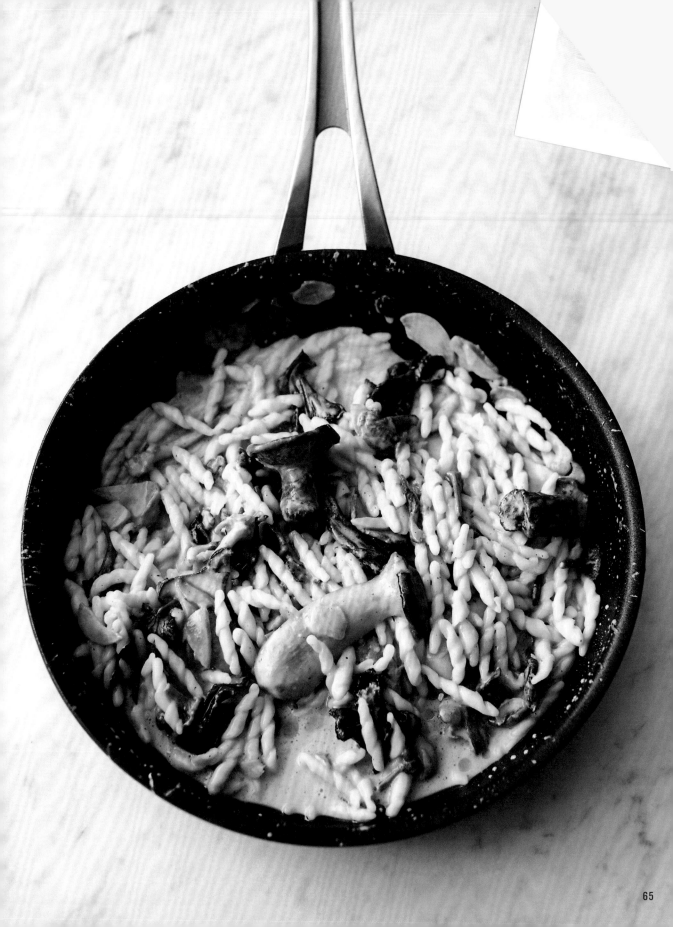

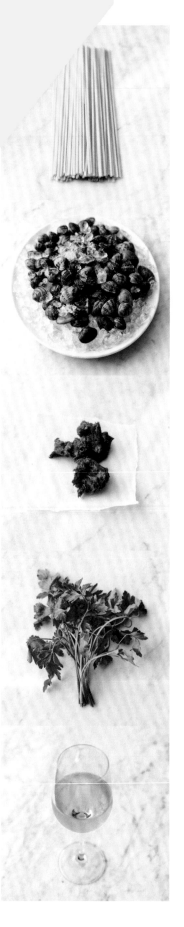

SPICY 'NDUJA VONGOLE

SERVES 2 | TOTAL JUST 15 MINUTES

150g dried linguine

500g clams, scrubbed

20g 'nduja

½ a bunch of fresh flat-leaf parsley (15g)

100ml light rosé wine

Cook the pasta in a pan of boiling salted water according to the packet instructions, draining 1 minute early and reserving a mugful of cooking water. Meanwhile, sort through the clams, giving any that aren't tightly closed a tap. If they don't close, discard them. Tear the 'nduja into a large cold non-stick frying pan, add 1 tablespoon of olive oil, place on a medium heat and let the 'nduja melt while you finely chop the parsley (stalks and all). Stir most of the parsley into the 'nduja pan with the clams and rosé, and put the lid on. After 3 or 4 minutes the clams will start to open – keep jiggling the pan until they've all opened, then remove from the heat, discarding any unopened clams.

Toss the drained pasta into the clam pan with a splash of reserved cooking water and simmer for 1 minute. Taste and season to perfection with sea salt and black pepper, if needed. Dish up, drizzle with a little extra virgin olive oil and scatter over the remaining parsley, and tuck in.

CALORIES	FAT	SAT FAT	PROTEIN	CARBS	SUGAR	SALT	FIBRE
556kcal	12.5g	2.1g	41.9g	62.5g	2.9g	0.6g	2.2g

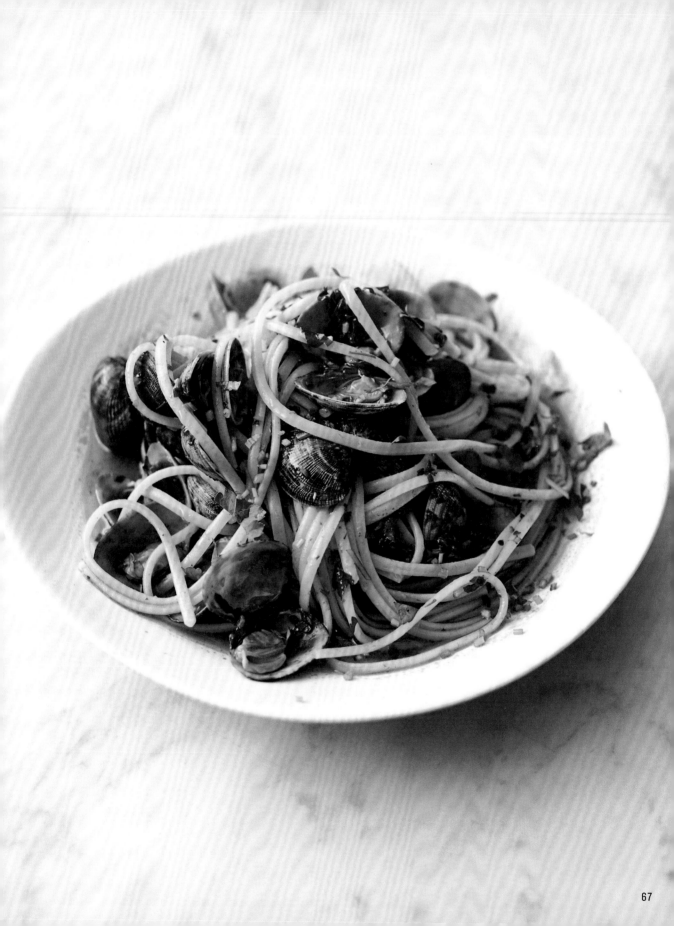

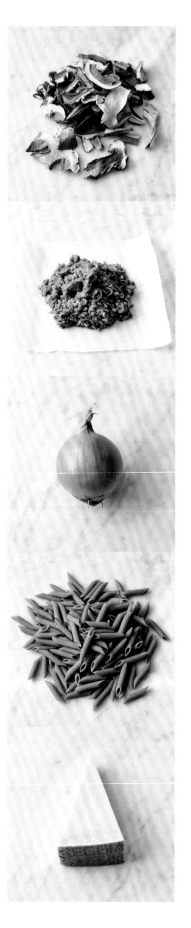

PORK PORCINI PASTA

SERVES 4   TOTAL 27 MINUTES

30g dried porcini mushrooms

300g minced pork shoulder

1 onion

300g dried wholewheat penne

50g Parmesan cheese

In a small bowl, cover the dried porcini with 400ml of boiling kettle water. Place the minced pork in a large shallow casserole pan with 1 tablespoon of olive oil, then break it up and fry on a high heat, stirring regularly. Meanwhile, peel and finely chop the onion, then the drained porcini, reserving the soaking water.

Stir the onion and porcini into the pan and fry for 10 minutes, or until golden. Add 1 tablespoon of red wine vinegar and the porcini water (discarding the last gritty bit). Simmer for 10 minutes on a low heat, while you cook the pasta in a pan of boiling salted water according to the packet instructions, draining 1 minute early and reserving a good mugful of cooking water.

Toss the drained pasta into the pork pan with 250ml of reserved cooking water, then finely grate in most of the Parmesan, taste and season to perfection with sea salt and black pepper. Toss over a low heat for 2 minutes to emulsify the sauce, then dish up. Finely grate over the remaining Parmesan, drizzle with a little extra virgin olive oil, and enjoy.

CALORIES	FAT	SAT FAT	PROTEIN	CARBS	SUGAR	SALT	FIBRE
524kcal	21.2g	7.2g	30.8g	55.9g	6.1g	0.6g	8.5g

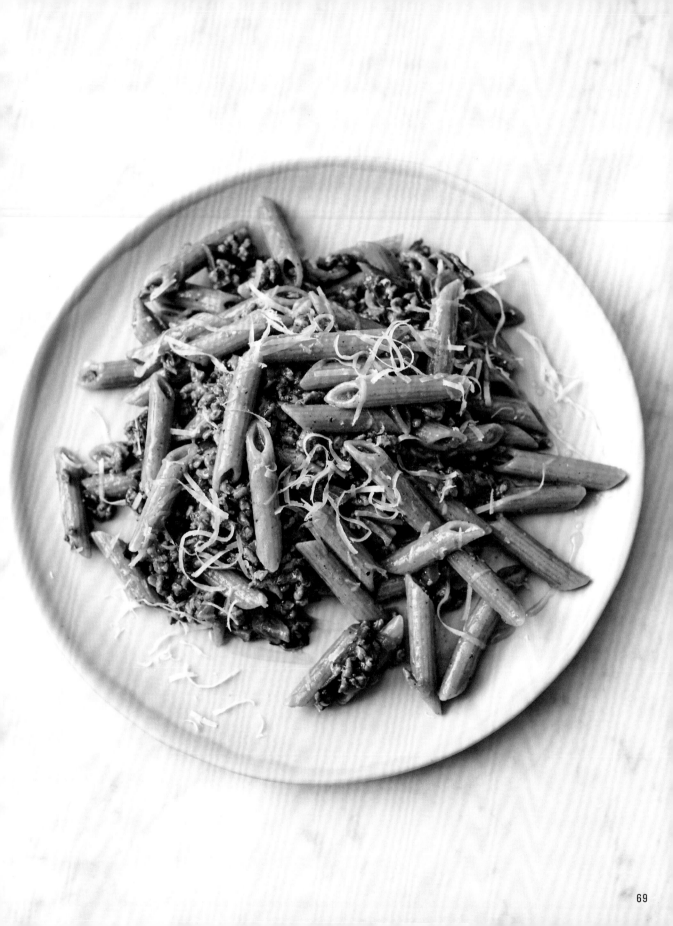

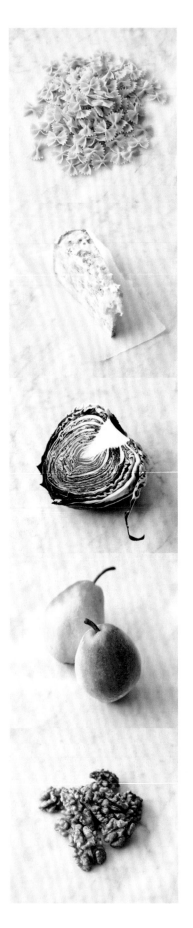

PEAR & GORGONZOLA FARFALLE

SERVES 2 | TOTAL JUST 15 MINUTES

150g dried farfalle

75g Gorgonzola cheese

½ a radicchio or 2 red chicory

2 super-ripe pears

30g shelled unsalted walnut halves

Cook the pasta in a medium pan of boiling salted water according to the packet instructions, then drain, reserving a mugful of cooking water. Melt the cheese in a heatproof bowl above the pasta as it cooks, removing carefully when gooey.

Meanwhile, slice the radicchio 1cm thick. Place it in a large dry non-stick frying pan on a high heat to char for 5 minutes, turning halfway. Peel the pears with a speed-peeler, then quarter, core and finely slice lengthways. Toss into the pan, crumble in most of the walnuts, add a splash of pasta cooking water, reduce to a medium heat and pop the lid on, then leave to caramelize slightly.

Toss the drained pasta and oozy Gorgonzola into the pear pan with a splash of red wine vinegar, and a splash of reserved cooking water, if needed. Taste, season to perfection with sea salt and black pepper, crumble over the remaining walnuts and drizzle with 1 teaspoon of extra virgin olive oil.

CALORIES	FAT	SAT FAT	PROTEIN	CARBS	SUGAR	SALT	FIBRE
575kcal	24.5g	8.5g	20.1g	73.2g	19.4g	1.3g	6.8g

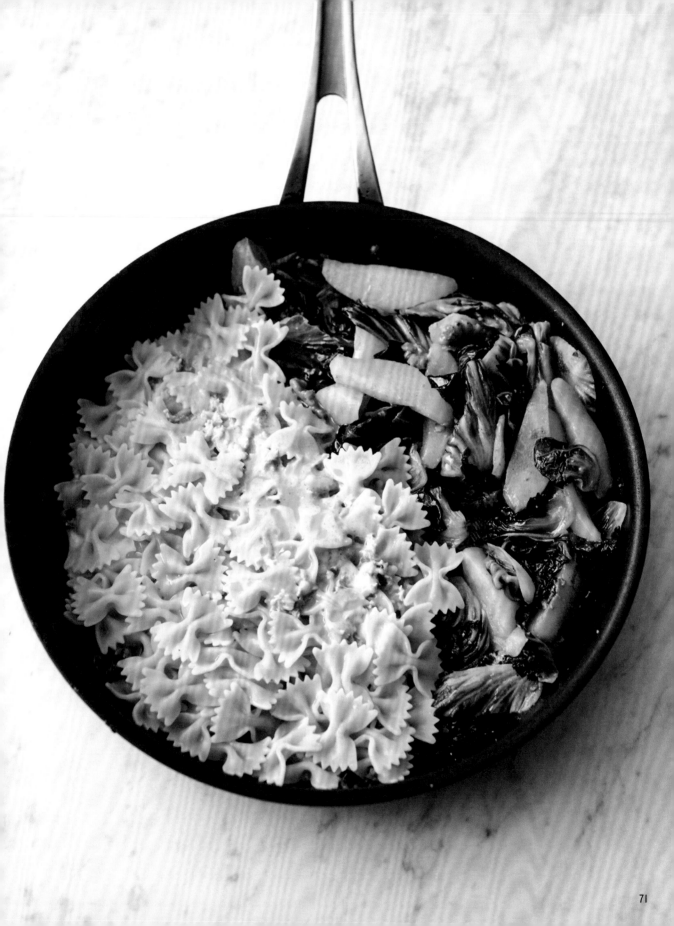

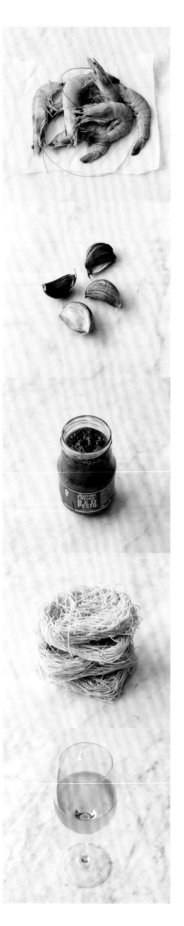

ROSÉ PESTO PRAWN PASTA

SERVES 2   TOTAL JUST 12 MINUTES

300g large raw shell-on king prawns

4 cloves of garlic

2 heaped teaspoons red pesto

150g dried taglierini or angel-hair pasta

150ml light rosé wine

Place 4 whole prawns in a large non-stick frying pan with 1 tablespoon of olive oil, off the heat. Pull off the rest of the prawn heads and chuck them into the pan for bonus flavour. Quickly pull the legs and tails off the prawns and peel off the shells. Run the tip of your knife down their backs and pull out the vein, then chop the prawns. Peel and finely slice the garlic. Put the frying pan on a medium-high heat and, after 2 minutes, stir in the garlic and chopped prawns, followed 1 minute later by the pesto, stirring regularly.

Meanwhile, cook the pasta in a pan of boiling salted water according to the packet instructions. Pour the rosé into the prawn pan and let it bubble and reduce for 1 minute. Drain the pasta, reserving a mugful of cooking water, then toss the pasta into the prawn pan, loosening with a little reserved cooking water, if needed. Toss over the heat for 1 minute, then taste, season to perfection with sea salt and black pepper, and dish up.

CALORIES	FAT	SAT FAT	PROTEIN	CARBS	SUGAR	SALT	FIBRE
468kcal	11.4g	1.6g	24.6g	58.2g	3.6g	0.6g	2.9g

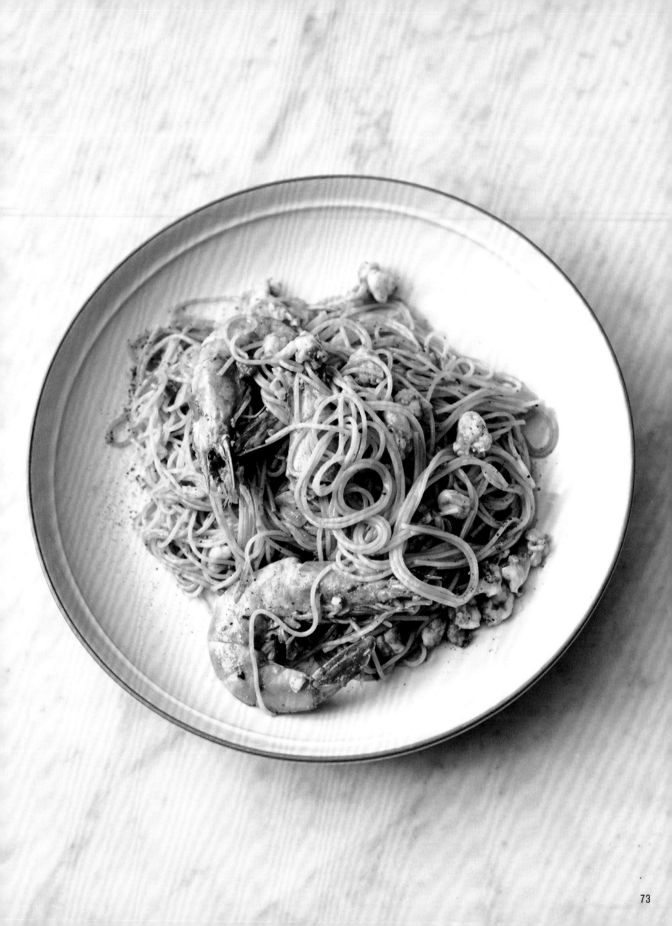

EGGS

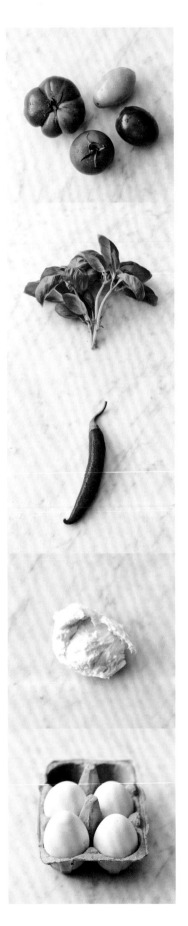

SCRAMBLED EGG OMELETTE

SERVES 2   TOTAL JUST 10 MINUTES

350g ripe mixed-colour tomatoes

½ a bunch of fresh basil (15g)

½–1 fresh red chilli

½ x 125g ball of mozzarella

4 large eggs

Finely slice the tomatoes, arrange over a sharing platter, then dress with a little extra virgin olive oil, red wine vinegar, sea salt and black pepper. Pick most of the basil leaves into a pestle and mortar, pound with a pinch of salt into a paste, then muddle in 1 tablespoon of extra virgin olive oil to make a basil oil.

Finely slice the chilli. Finely chop the mozzarella. Place a 26cm non-stick frying pan on a medium heat with ½ a tablespoon of olive oil. Beat and pour in the eggs, then stir regularly with a rubber spatula, moving the eggs gently around the pan. When they're lightly scrambled but still loose, stop stirring and scatter the mozzarella in the centre, then drizzle over the basil oil. Let the bottom of the eggs set for 1 minute, then – technique time – pick up the pan, tilt it down and, with your other hand, keep tapping your wrist until it shakes the eggs up the side of the pan; use the spatula to flip it back to the middle, then fold the top half back over, too. Turn it upside down on to the tomato platter, set side up.

Slice down the centre to reveal the oozy scrambled eggs in the middle. Scatter over the chilli (as much as you dare!) and remaining basil leaves, and tuck on in.

CALORIES	FAT	SAT FAT	PROTEIN	CARBS	SUGAR	SALT	FIBRE
356kcal	28.9g	9g	20.9g	4.4g	4g	1.2g	1.3g

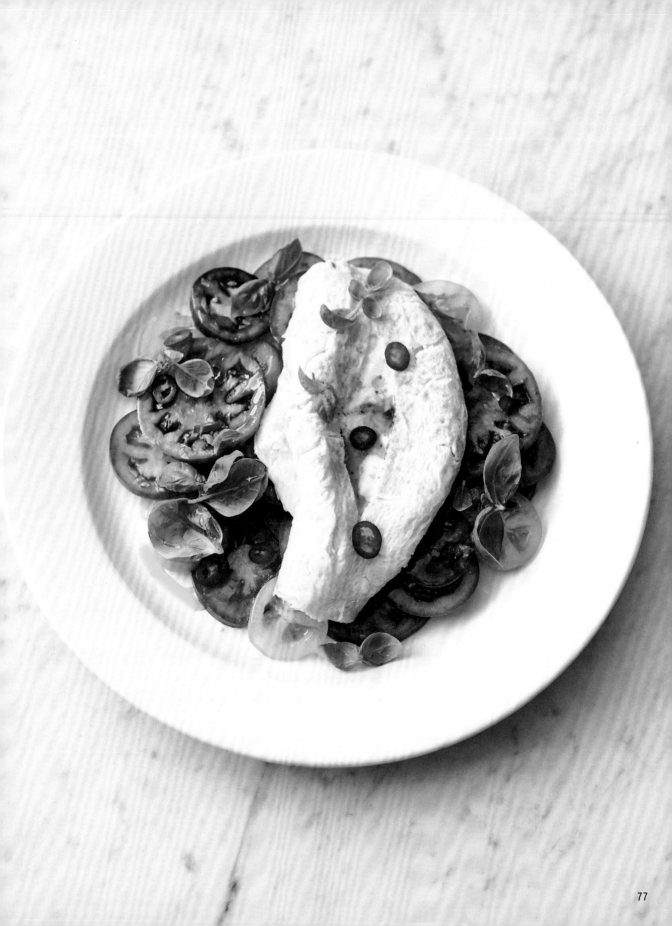

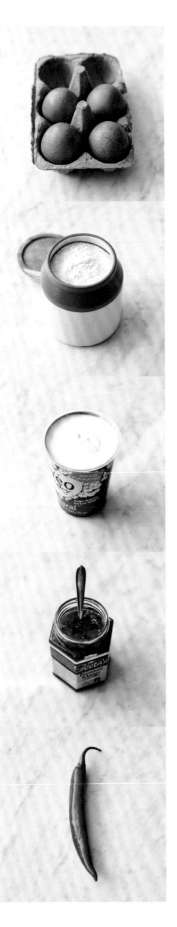

EGG & MANGO CHUTNEY FLATBREADS

SERVES 2 | TOTAL JUST 12 MINUTES

4 large eggs

100g self-raising flour, plus extra for dusting

6 tablespoons natural yoghurt

2 tablespoons mango chutney

1 fresh red chilli

Lower the eggs into a pan of vigorously simmering water and boil for 5½ minutes exactly, then refresh under cold water until cool enough to handle, and peel. Meanwhile, put a large non-stick frying pan on a medium-high heat. In a bowl, mix the flour with a little pinch of sea salt, 4 tablespoons of yoghurt and 1 tablespoon of olive oil until you have a dough. Halve, then roll out each piece on a flour-dusted surface until just under ½cm thick. Cook for 3 minutes, or until golden, turning halfway.

Dot the mango chutney and remaining yoghurt over the breads. Halve the soft-boiled eggs and arrange on top, smashing them in with a fork, if you like. Finely slice the chilli and scatter over (as much as you dare!), drizzle with a little extra virgin olive oil and season with salt and black pepper from a height.

CALORIES	FAT	SAT FAT	PROTEIN	CARBS	SUGAR	SALT	FIBRE
524kcal	24.6g	7.6g	24.4g	55.6g	17.9g	2g	1.5g

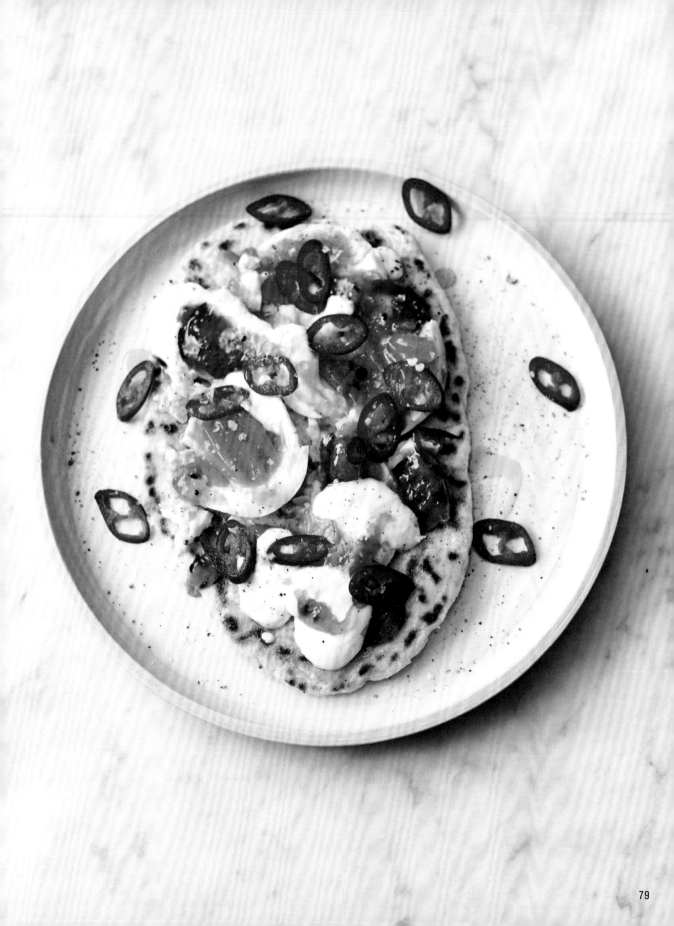

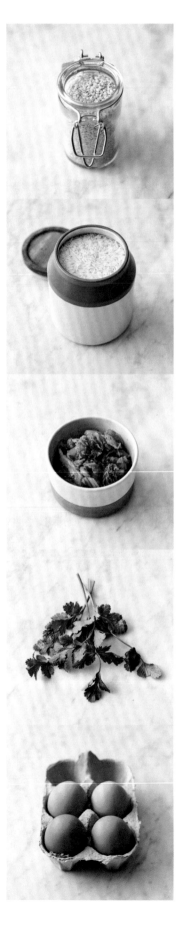

KOREAN EGGS & RICE

SERVES 2 | TOTAL 22 MINUTES

1 heaped tablespoon sesame seeds

150g basmati rice

150g kimchee

4 sprigs of fresh coriander

4 large eggs

Toast the sesame seeds in a dry 26cm non-stick frying pan on a medium heat. Once lightly golden, remove to a plate, reducing the heat to medium-low. Place the rice in the pan with a small pinch of sea salt, then pour in 400ml of water. Cover and cook for 10 minutes, or until the rice has absorbed all the liquid.

Finely chop the kimchee with half the coriander leaves, beat in the eggs, then pour over the rice, spreading it out evenly with a spatula. Cover and leave for another 5 to 10 minutes, or until the eggs are just set.

Loosen the edges with a spatula, then slide it out on to a plate – I like to fold one half back on itself to expose the underside. Scatter over the toasted sesame seeds, pick over the remaining coriander leaves, then tuck on in.

CALORIES	FAT	SAT FAT	PROTEIN	CARBS	SUGAR	SALT	FIBRE
477kcal	15.7g	3.9g	22.5g	65.6g	0.8g	1.5g	2.2g

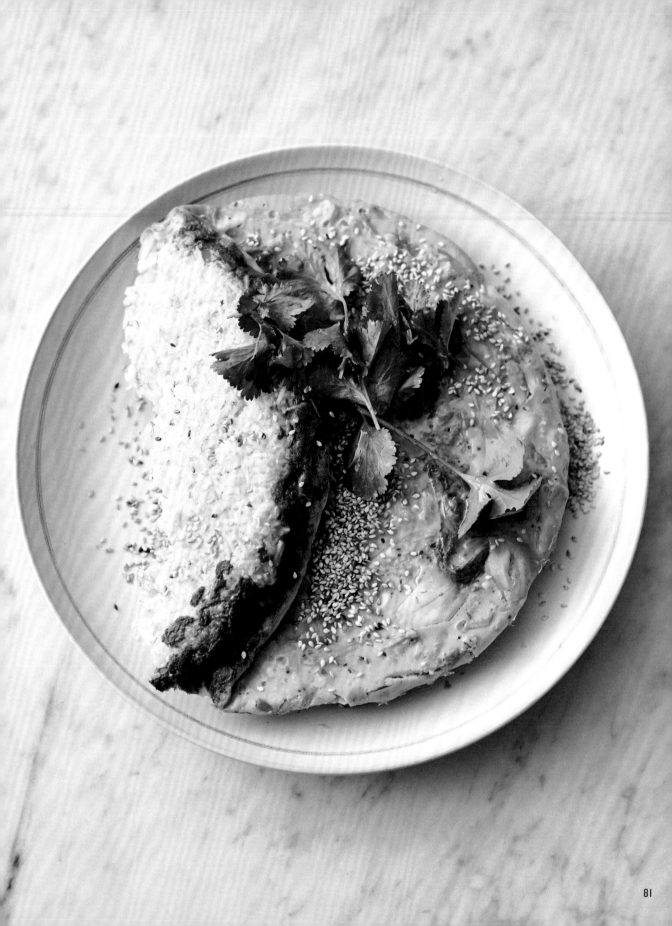

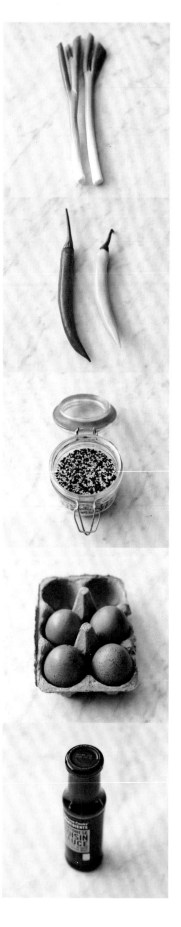

ASIAN FRIED EGGS

SERVES 2 | TOTAL JUST 10 MINUTES

2 spring onions

1–2 fresh mixed-colour chillies

2 heaped tablespoons mixed sesame seeds

4 large eggs

2 tablespoons hoisin sauce

Trim the spring onions, very finely slice at an angle with the chillies, pop both into a bowl of ice-cold water, add a swig of red wine vinegar and put aside.

Place a large non-stick frying pan on a medium-high heat and lightly toast the sesame seeds for 1 minute. Drizzle in 1 tablespoon of olive oil, then crack in the eggs. Put a lid on the pan, and fry to your liking.

Place the eggs on your plates – I like one facing up and one facing down. From a height, drizzle over the hoisin (loosening with a splash of water first, if needed). Drain and scatter over the spring onions and chillies, stab the yolks, and enjoy.

CALORIES	FAT	SAT FAT	PROTEIN	CARBS	SUGAR	SALT	FIBRE
350kcal	27.9g	5.9g	17.6g	8.3g	7.4g	1g	1.7g

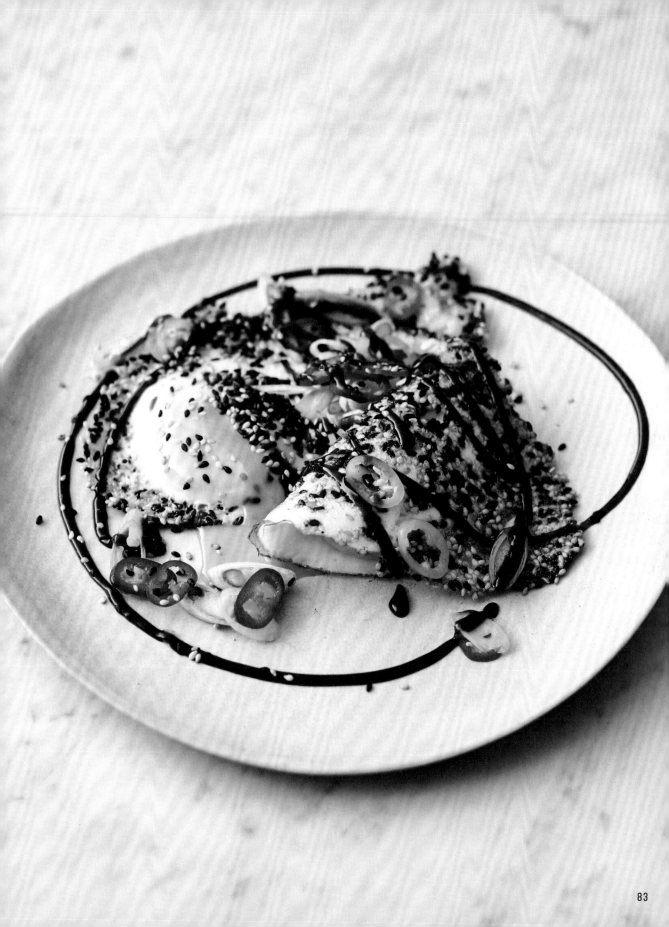

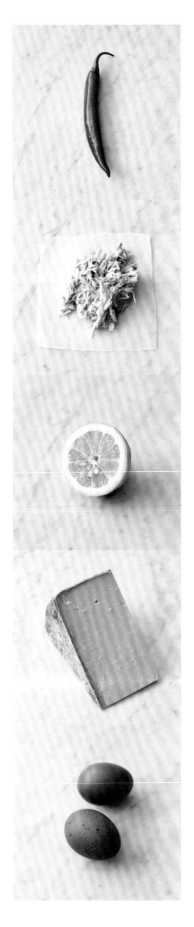

CHILLI CRAB SILKY OMELETTE

SERVES 1   TOTAL JUST 10 MINUTES

½–1 fresh red chilli

75g mixed brown & white crabmeat

½ a lemon

10g Cheddar cheese

2 large eggs

Deseed and finely chop the chilli. Mix as much as you dare with the crabmeat, a squeeze of lemon juice and a little sea salt and black pepper. Finely grate the cheese. Beat the eggs well, ready to go.

Get a 30cm non-stick frying pan nice and hot on a medium-high heat, then add a drizzle of olive oil and wipe it around and out with a ball of kitchen paper. Pour in the eggs, swirling them around the pan and up the sides. Working quickly, sprinkle over the cheese from a height, followed by the dressed crab, then turn the heat off. Use a rubber spatula to gently ease it away from the edges and quickly roll it up a few times – you want to create layers, so how you roll and whether it tears doesn't matter, just don't overcook it. Turn the omelette out on to a plate, drizzle with a little extra virgin olive oil, and tuck in.

CALORIES	FAT	SAT FAT	PROTEIN	CARBS	SUGAR	SALT	FIBRE
300kcal	19.1g	6.6g	30.6g	2.8g	0.9g	2g	0.5g

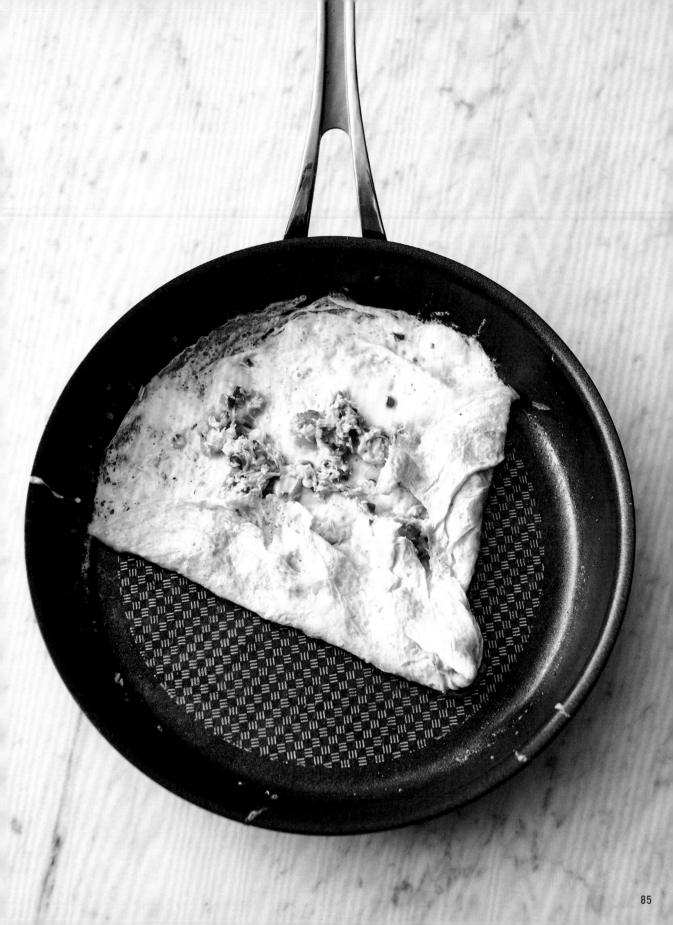

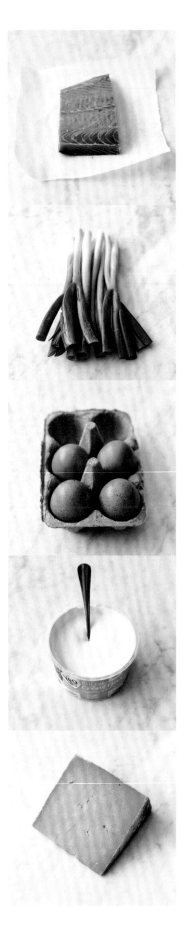

HOT-SMOKED SALMON FRITTATA

SERVES 2 | TOTAL JUST 13 MINUTES

125g hot-smoked salmon, skin off

1 bunch of spring onions

4 large eggs

2 heaped tablespoons half-fat crème fraîche

40g Red Leicester cheese

Preheat the grill to high. Place a 26cm non-stick ovenproof frying pan on a medium-high heat. Put the salmon into the pan, breaking it up as it starts to sizzle. Trim, finely slice and add the spring onions, along with a pinch of black pepper. Stir occasionally for 5 minutes while, in a large bowl, you vigorously whisk the eggs until they've doubled in size.

Reduce the heat to low, stir in the crème fraîche and grate in the cheese. Pour the contents of the pan into the egg bowl, mix well, then pour back into the pan, swirling it around and up the sides. Grill for 5 minutes, or until golden, set and just cooked through – keep an eye on it. Loosen the edges with a spatula, then slide on to a board, slice, and serve.

CALORIES	FAT	SAT FAT	PROTEIN	CARBS	SUGAR	SALT	FIBRE
420kcal	29.4g	11.8g	36.8g	3.7g	3.1g	2.1g	0g

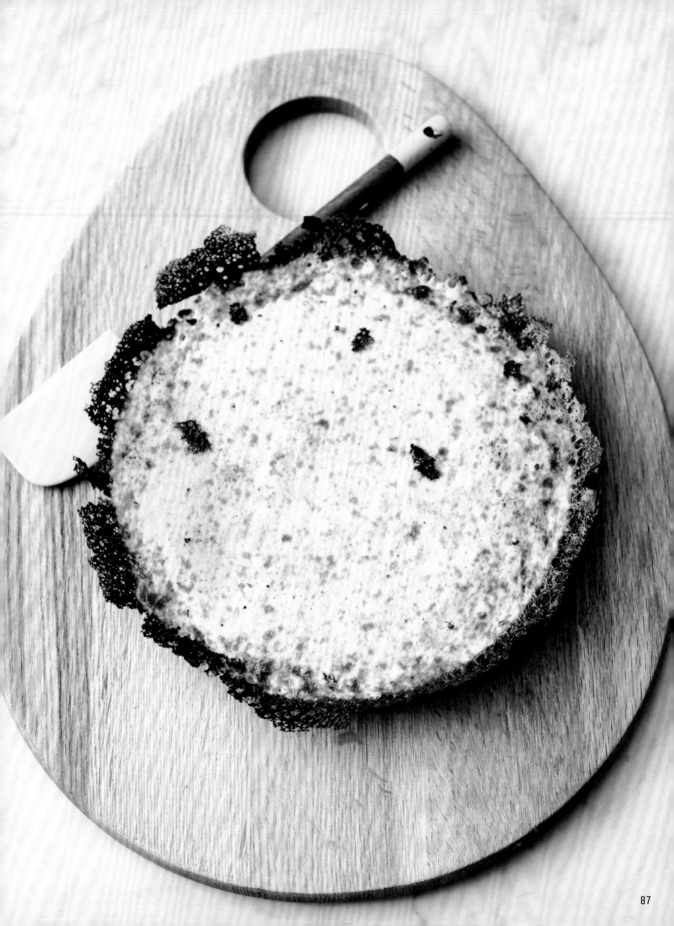

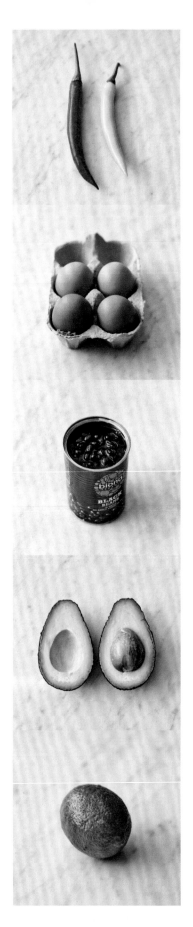

ALL-DAY MEXICAN BREAKFAST

SERVES 2   TOTAL JUST 15 MINUTES

1–2 fresh mixed-colour chillies

4 large eggs

1 x 400g tin of black beans

1 ripe avocado

1 lime

Finely slice the chillies (use as much as you dare!). Sprinkle half of them into a 30cm non-stick frying pan on a medium heat with 1 teaspoon of olive oil. Once they start to sizzle, evenly crack in the eggs, then spoon the black beans and just half the juice from the tin in and around the eggs. Season with sea salt and black pepper, cover and cook the eggs to your liking.

Meanwhile, halve, peel and destone the avocado, slice into thin wedges, dress with the lime juice and season to perfection. Arrange the avocado around the pan, scatter over the rest of the chillies, stab the egg yolks, and dish up.

CALORIES	FAT	SAT FAT	PROTEIN	CARBS	SUGAR	SALT	FIBRE
381kcal	24.8g	5.8g	23.8g	11.1g	1.2g	0.9g	12.1g

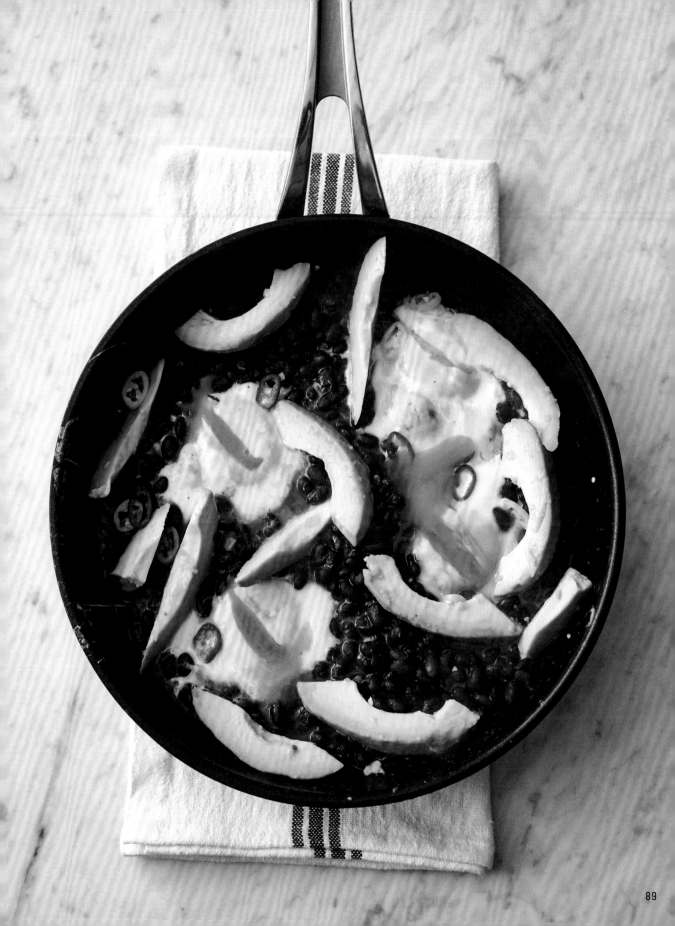

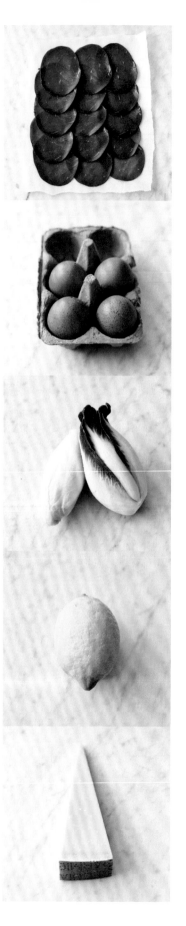

EGG RIBBON SALAD

SERVES 2 | TOTAL JUST 15 MINUTES

50g finely sliced bresaola

4 large eggs

2 mixed-colour chicory

1 lemon

10g Parmesan cheese

Arrange the bresaola slices on your plates. Beat the eggs well. Get a 26cm non-stick frying pan nice and hot on a medium heat, then add a drizzle of olive oil and wipe it around and out with a ball of kitchen paper. Pour in just enough egg to thinly cover the base of the pan, swirling it up around the sides and pouring any excess back into your bowl, almost like an egg pancake. As soon as it's set, use a rubber spatula to ease it away at the sides, and out on to a board. Repeat with the remaining egg. Cool, roll up and finely slice.

Trim and finely slice the chicory. Dress with the lemon juice and ½ a tablespoon of extra virgin olive oil, then toss with the egg ribbons, taste and season to perfection with sea salt and black pepper. Pile in the centre of the bresaola, shave over the Parmesan, then finish with a little extra virgin olive oil.

CALORIES	FAT	SAT FAT	PROTEIN	CARBS	SUGAR	SALT	FIBRE
280kcal	19.5g	5.7g	26.3g	2.9g	0.9g	1.3g	0g

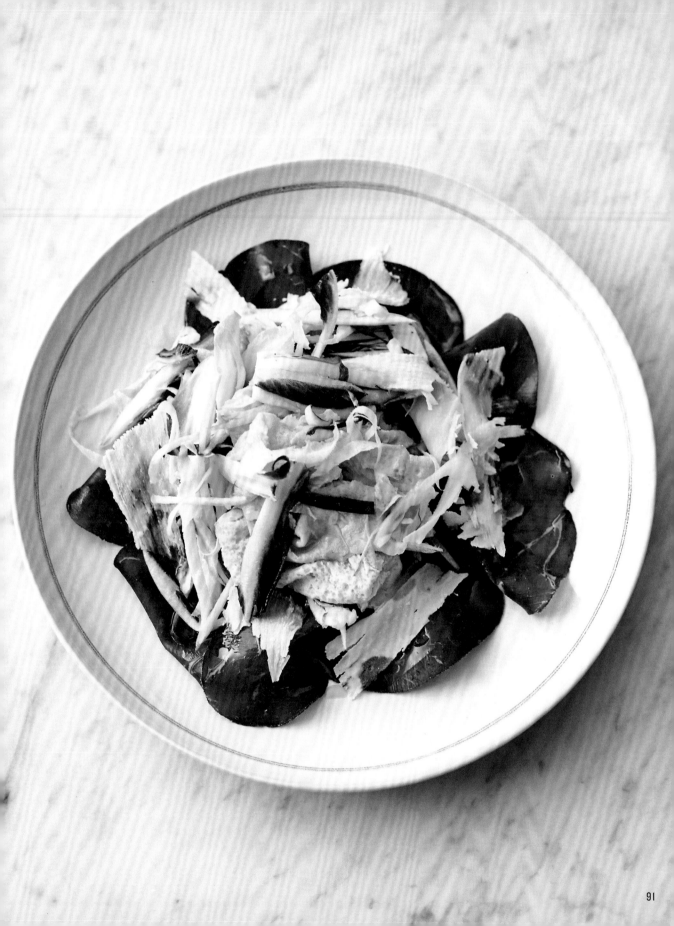

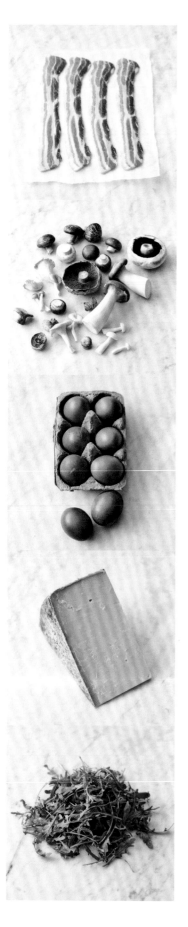

SMOKY MUSHROOM FRITTATA

SERVES 4   TOTAL 24 MINUTES

4 rashers of smoked streaky bacon

400g mixed mushrooms

8 large eggs

80g Cheddar cheese

50g rocket

Preheat the oven to 200°C/400°F/gas 6. Slice the bacon and fry in 1 teaspoon of olive oil in a 26cm non-stick ovenproof frying pan on a medium heat for 2 minutes. Add the mushrooms, tearing up any larger ones. Season with sea salt and black pepper, then fry for 5 minutes, or until golden, tossing regularly.

Lightly beat the eggs, then pour into the pan and bomb over nuggets of cheese. Transfer to the oven for 10 minutes, or until nicely set. Loosen the edges with a spatula, then slide on to a board. Dress the rocket in a little extra virgin olive oil and red wine vinegar, and sprinkle on top.

CALORIES	FAT	SAT FAT	PROTEIN	CARBS	SUGAR	SALT	FIBRE
299kcal	23.5g	8.7g	22.9g	0.4g	0.2g	1.5g	1.3g

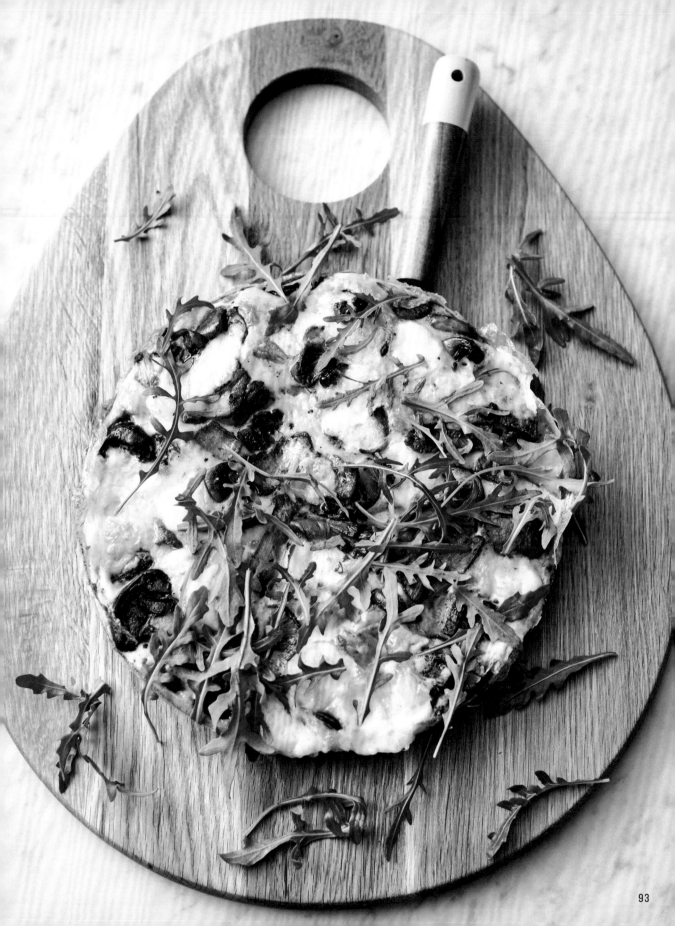

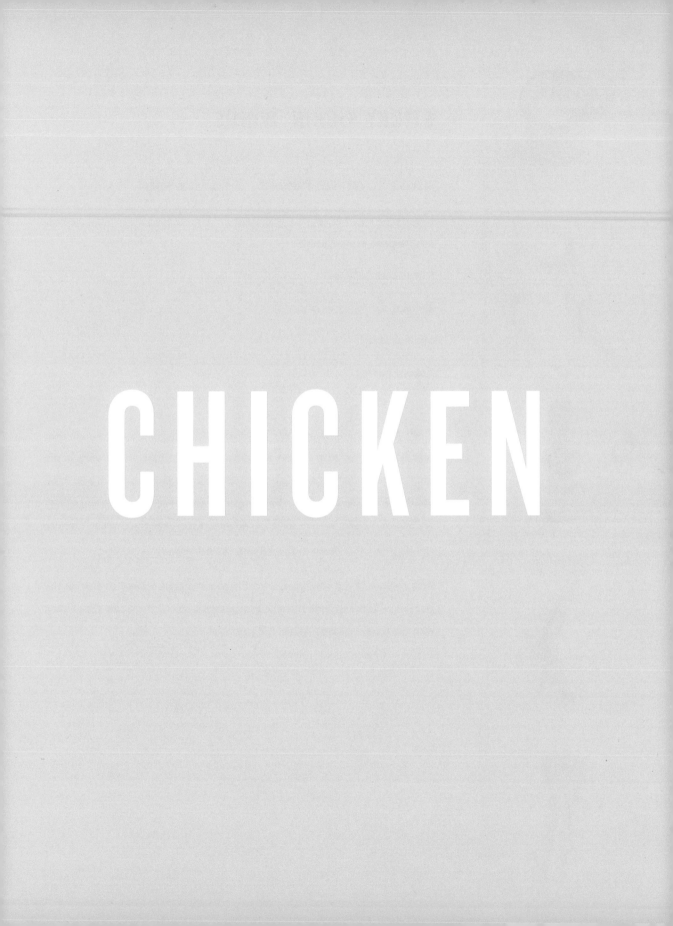

CHICKEN

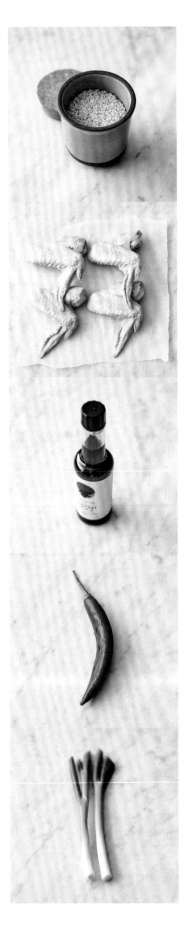

STICKY KICKIN' WINGS

SERVES 2   FAST PREP 6 MINUTES   COOK 40 MINUTES

1 tablespoon sesame seeds

4 large chicken wings

2 tablespoons teriyaki sauce

1 fresh red chilli

2 spring onions

Toast the sesame seeds in a dry 20cm non-stick frying pan on a medium heat until lightly golden, then remove to a plate. Still on the heat, sit the wings in the pan – they should fit snugly. Let them colour for 1 minute on each side, then add the teriyaki and just cover the wings with water. Halve the chilli lengthways and add to the pan. Simmer for 35 to 40 minutes, or until the chicken is tender and the sauce is nice and sticky, turning occasionally.

Add a splash of red wine vinegar to the pan and jiggle around to pick up the gnarly bits. Trim and finely slice the spring onions, scatter them over the chicken with the toasted sesame seeds, and get stuck in.

CALORIES	FAT	SAT FAT	PROTEIN	CARBS	SUGAR	SALT	FIBRE
306kcal	18.6g	4.9g	27.1g	7.4g	6.2g	1.4g	0g

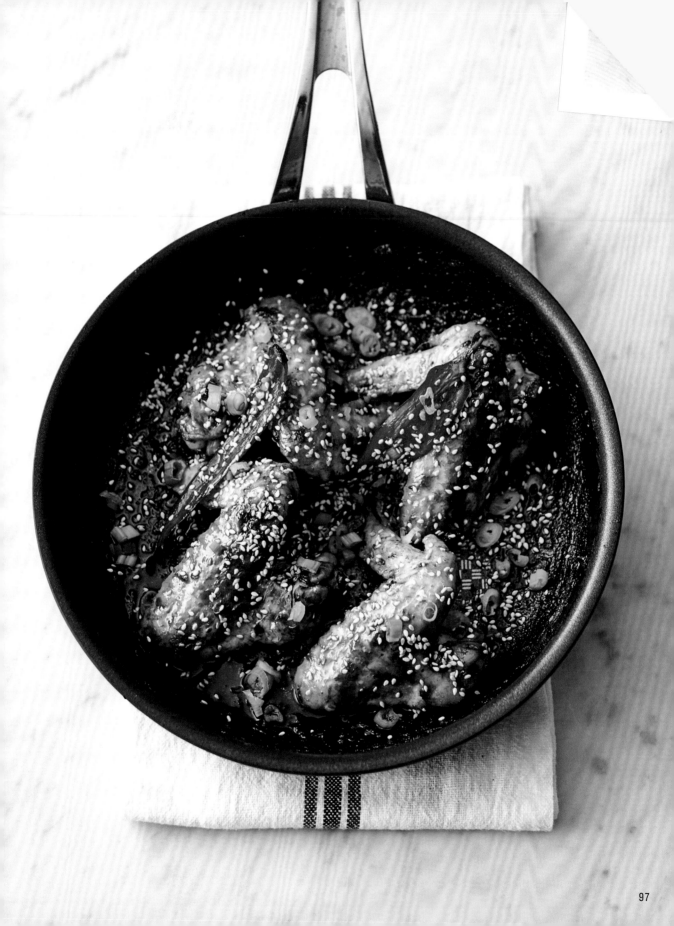

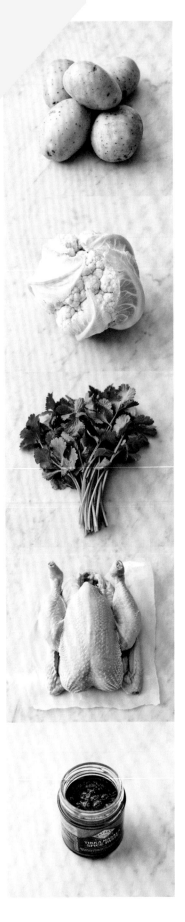

ROAST TIKKA CHICKEN

SERVES 4 | FAST PREP 10 MINUTES | SLOW COOK 1 HOUR

800g potatoes

1 small head of cauliflower (600g)

1 bunch of fresh coriander (30g)

1 x 1.2kg whole chicken

2 tablespoons tikka curry paste

Preheat the oven to 180°C/350°F/gas 4. Wash the potatoes and chop into 3cm chunks. Trim the cauli stalk, remove any tough outer leaves, then chop the cauli and nice leaves the same size as the spuds. Finely slice the coriander stalks (reserving the leaves in a bowl of cold water). In a 30cm x 40cm roasting tray, toss the veg and coriander stalks with a pinch of sea salt and black pepper, and 1 tablespoon each of olive oil and red wine vinegar.

Sit the chicken in the tray and rub all over with the tikka paste, getting into all the nooks and crannies. Place the chicken directly on the bars of the oven, scrunch everything in the tray and place exactly underneath the chicken to catch the tasty juices. Roast for 1 hour, or until everything is golden and cooked through, turning the veg halfway. Sit the chicken on top of the veg to rest for 5 minutes, then sprinkle over the drained coriander leaves and serve, tossing the veg in all the tasty juices before dishing up.

CALORIES	FAT	SAT FAT	PROTEIN	CARBS	SUGAR	SALT	FIBRE
467kcal	15.9g	3.3g	42.3g	40.6g	5.7g	1.1g	5.9g

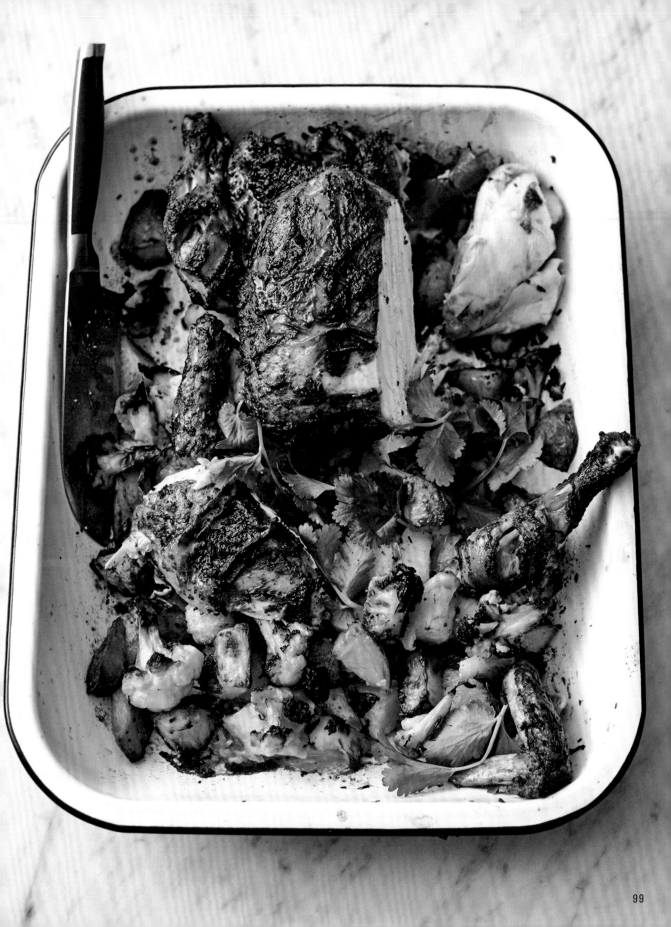

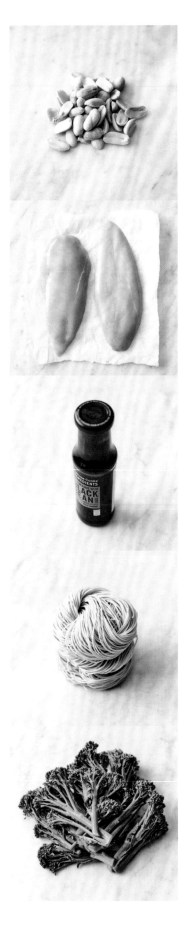

CHICKEN NOODLE STIR-FRY

SERVES 2   TOTAL 16 MINUTES

30g unsalted peanuts

2 x 120g skinless chicken breasts

2 tablespoons black bean sauce

150g medium egg noodles

200g tenderstem broccoli

Place a large non-stick frying pan on a medium heat and toast the peanuts as it heats up, tossing regularly, then remove and set aside, leaving the pan on the heat. Meanwhile, score the chicken lengthways at 1cm intervals, going about halfway through. In a bowl, toss the chicken with 1 tablespoon each of olive oil, red wine vinegar and black bean sauce to coat. Cook in the hot pan for 3 minutes on each side, or until dark, gnarly and cooked through.

Cook the noodles in a large pan of boiling salted water according to the packet instructions. Trim the broccoli (halving any thick stalks lengthways) and add to the water for the last 2 minutes. Remove the chicken to a board. Use tongs to carefully drag the just-cooked noodles and broccoli with a bit of their water straight into the frying pan. Pound half the peanuts in a pestle and mortar until fine, toss into the pan with the remaining black bean sauce until well mixed, then divide between your plates. Slice the chicken and place on top, scatter over the remaining peanuts, drizzle with a little extra virgin olive oil, and dig in.

CALORIES	FAT	SAT FAT	PROTEIN	CARBS	SUGAR	SALT	FIBRE
579kcal	18.7g	3.4g	45.5g	60.7g	5.5g	1.4g	4.3g

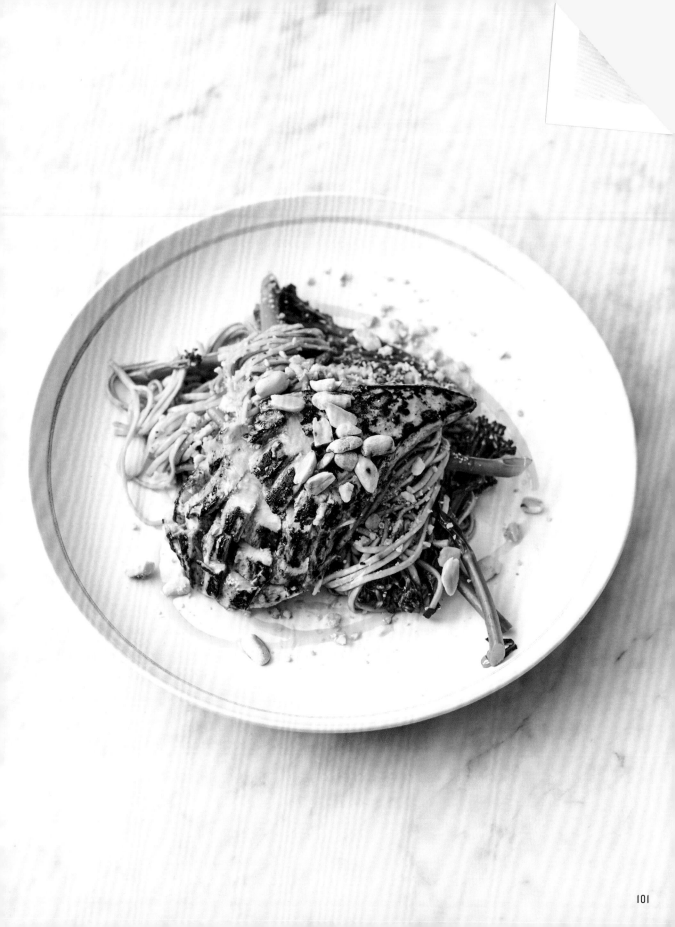

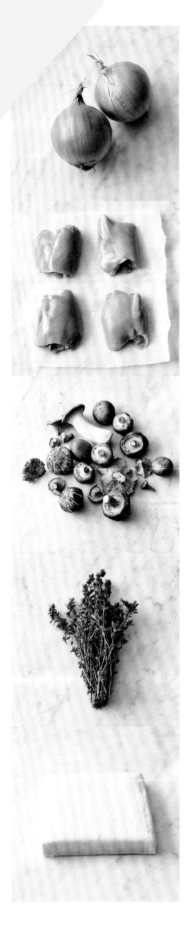

CHICKEN POT PIE

SERVES 4   TOTAL 30 MINUTES

2 onions

600g chicken thighs, skin off, bone out

350g mixed mushrooms

1 bunch of fresh thyme (30g)

375g block of all-butter puff pastry (cold)

Preheat the oven to 220°C/425°F/gas 7. Place a 30cm non-stick ovenproof frying pan on a high heat, with a smaller non-stick pan on a medium heat alongside. Pour 1 tablespoon of olive oil into the larger pan. Peel and roughly chop the onions, adding them to the larger pan as you go. Roughly chop two-thirds of the thighs, finely chop the rest, and add to the onion pan. Cook for 6 minutes, or until golden, stirring occasionally. Meanwhile, place the mushrooms in the dry pan, tearing up any larger ones. Let them toast and get nutty for 4 minutes, then tip into the chicken pan and strip in half the thyme leaves.

Remove the pan from the heat, add a pinch of sea salt and black pepper, then stir in 1 tablespoon of red wine vinegar and 150ml of water. Working quickly, roll out the pastry so it's 2cm bigger than the pan, then place it over the filling, using a wooden spoon to push it into the edges. Very lightly criss-cross the pastry, then brush with 1 teaspoon of olive oil. Poke the remaining thyme sprigs into the middle of the pie. Bake at the bottom of the oven for 15 minutes, or until golden and puffed up. Easy!

CALORIES	FAT	SAT FAT	PROTEIN	CARBS	SUGAR	SALT	FIBRE
683kcal	40.7g	19.8g	36.7g	42g	7.2g	1.2g	4.3g

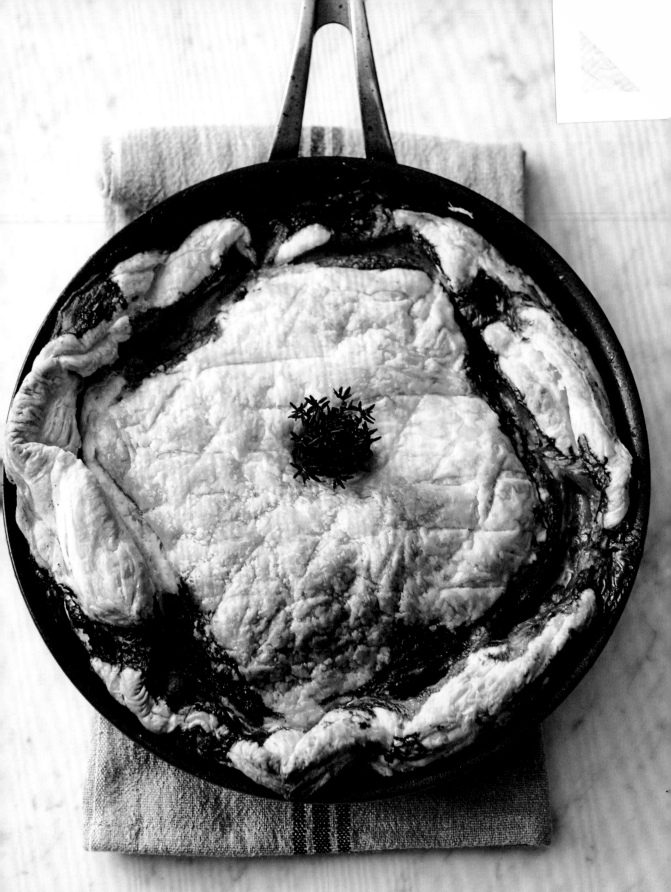

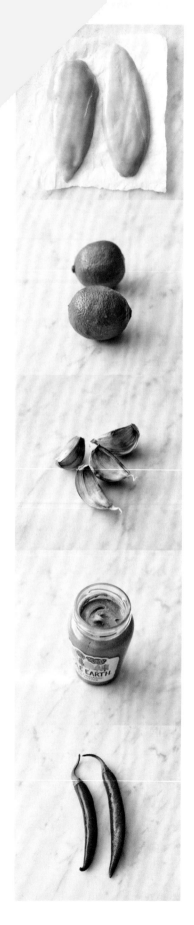

GNARLY PEANUT CHICKEN

SERVES 2   TOTAL JUST 12 MINUTES

2 x 120g skinless chicken breasts

2 limes

4 cloves of garlic

2 heaped tablespoons peanut butter

1–2 fresh red chillies

Turn the grill on to medium-high. Score the chicken breasts in a criss-cross fashion, rub with 1 tablespoon of olive oil, a pinch of sea salt and black pepper and the finely grated zest of 1 lime. Place criss-cross side down in a cold 26cm non-stick ovenproof frying pan and put it on a medium-high heat, while you peel and finely grate the garlic into a bowl. Squeeze in the juice from 1½ limes, stir in the peanut butter and loosen with enough water to give you a spoonable consistency. Finely slice the chilli, then mix (as much as you dare!) through the sauce, taste and season to perfection.

Flip the chicken over, spoon over the sauce, then transfer to the grill, roughly 10cm from the heat, for 5 minutes, or until gnarly and cooked through. Finely grate over the remaining lime zest, then drizzle with 1 teaspoon of extra virgin olive oil. Serve with lime wedges, for squeezing over.

CALORIES	FAT	SAT FAT	PROTEIN	CARBS	SUGAR	SALT	FIBRE
405kcal	25g	4.6g	38.6g	6g	1.8g	0.9g	1.8g

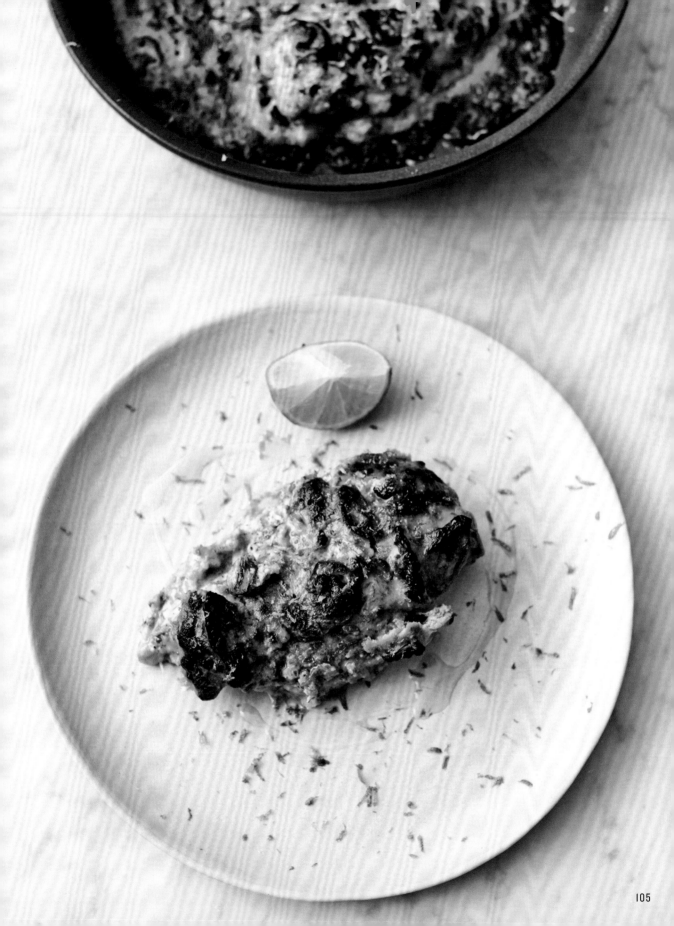

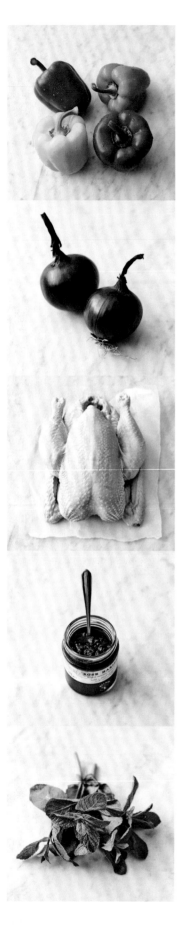

HARISSA CHICKEN TRAYBAKE

SERVES 4　｜　FAST PREP 9 MINUTES　｜　COOK 50 MINUTES

4 mixed-colour peppers

2 red onions

1 x 1.2kg whole chicken

4 heaped teaspoons rose harissa

4 sprigs of fresh mint

Preheat the oven to 180°C/350°F/gas 4. Deseed the peppers and tear into big chunks, peel and quarter the onions and break apart into petals, then place it all in a 30cm x 40cm roasting tray. Use a large sharp knife to carefully cut down the back of the chicken, so you can open it out flat, then score the legs. Add to the tray with the harissa, and a little sea salt, black pepper and red wine vinegar. Toss well, making sure you get into all the nooks and crannies of the chicken.

Sit the chicken flat on top of the veg, skin side up, and roast it all for 50 minutes, or until gnarly and cooked through. Pick over the mint leaves before dishing up.

CALORIES	FAT	SAT FAT	PROTEIN	CARBS	SUGAR	SALT	FIBRE
297kcal	11.4g	2.7g	35g	13.9g	12.2g	0.9g	5.8g

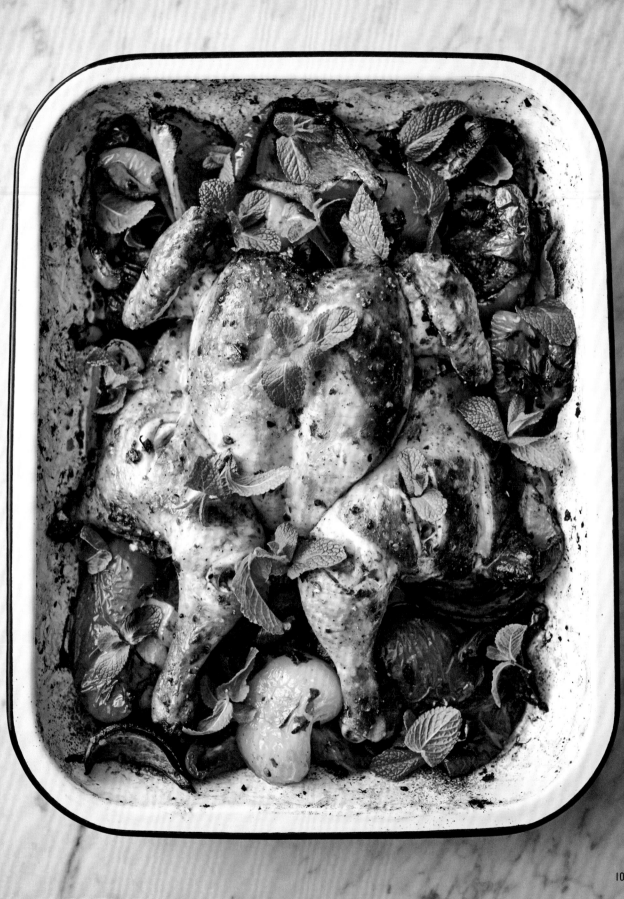

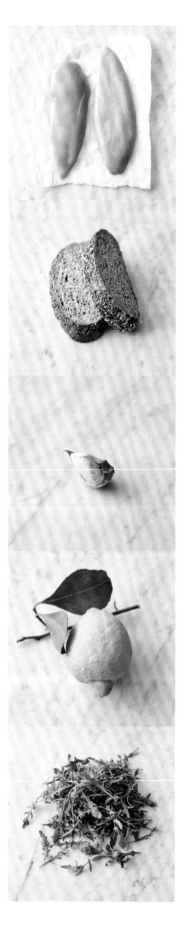

CRISPY GARLICKY CHICKEN

SERVES 2   TOTAL 20 MINUTES

2 x 120g skinless chicken breasts

2 thick slices of seeded wholemeal bread (75g each)

1 clove of garlic

1 lemon

50g rocket

Place the chicken breasts between two large sheets of greaseproof paper, and whack with the base of a large non-stick frying pan to flatten them to about 1cm thick. Tear the bread into a food processor, then peel, chop and add the garlic, and blitz into fairly fine crumbs. Pour the crumbs over the chicken, roughly pat on to each side, then re-cover with the paper and whack again, to hammer the crumbs into the chicken and flatten them further.

Put the pan on a medium heat. Fry the crumbed chicken in 1 tablespoon of olive oil for 3 minutes on each side, or until crisp, golden and cooked through. Slice, plate up, season to perfection with sea salt and black pepper, sprinkle with lemon-dressed rocket, and serve with lemon wedges, for squeezing over.

CALORIES	FAT	SAT FAT	PROTEIN	CARBS	SUGAR	SALT	FIBRE
366kcal	11g	2g	36.6g	32.1g	2.4g	1.1g	5.8g

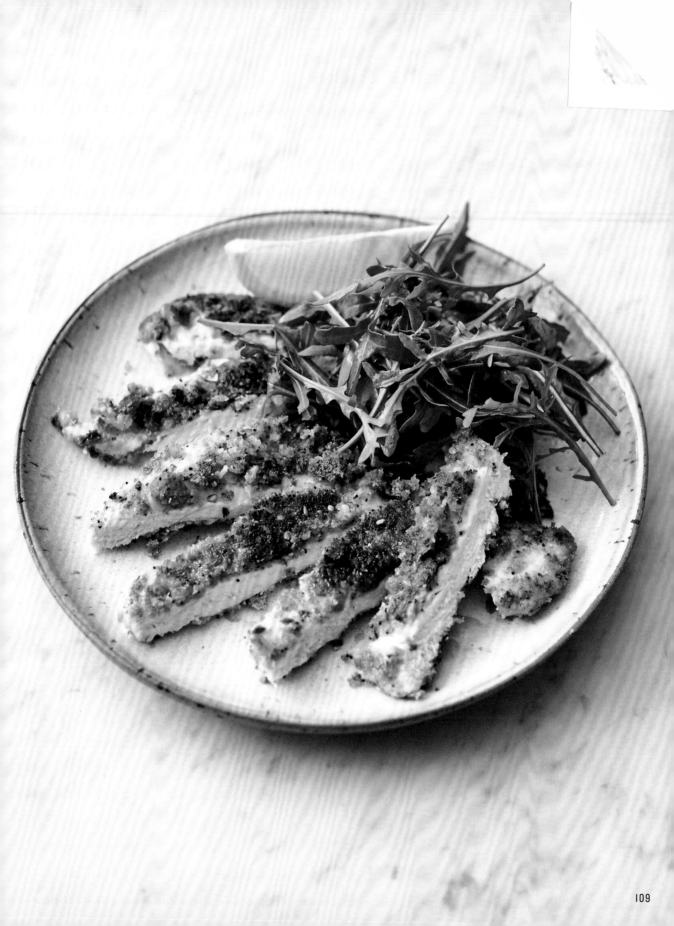

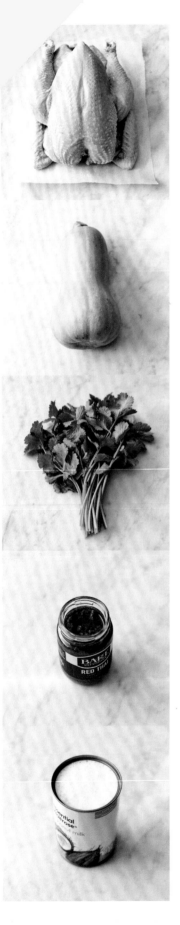

THAI RED CHICKEN SOUP

SERVES 6   FAST PREP 10 MINUTES   SLOW COOK 1 HOUR 20 MINUTES

1 x 1.6kg whole chicken

1 butternut squash (1.2kg)

1 bunch of fresh coriander (30g)

100g Thai red curry paste

1 x 400ml tin of light coconut milk

Sit the chicken in a large, deep pan. Carefully halve the squash lengthways, then cut into 3cm chunks, discarding the seeds. Slice the coriander stalks, add to the pan with the squash, curry paste and coconut milk, then pour in 1 litre of water. Cover and simmer on a medium heat for 1 hour 20 minutes.

Use tongs to remove the chicken to a platter. Spoon any fat from the surface of the soup over the chicken, then sprinkle with half the coriander leaves. Serve with 2 forks for divvying up the meat at the table. Use a potato masher to crush some of the squash, giving your soup a thicker texture. Taste, season to perfection with sea salt and black pepper, then divide between six bowls and sprinkle with the remaining coriander. Shred and add chicken, as you dig in.

CALORIES	FAT	SAT FAT	PROTEIN	CARBS	SUGAR	SALT	FIBRE
354kcal	16.1g	5.8g	32.8g	20.5g	11.8g	0.9g	4.8g

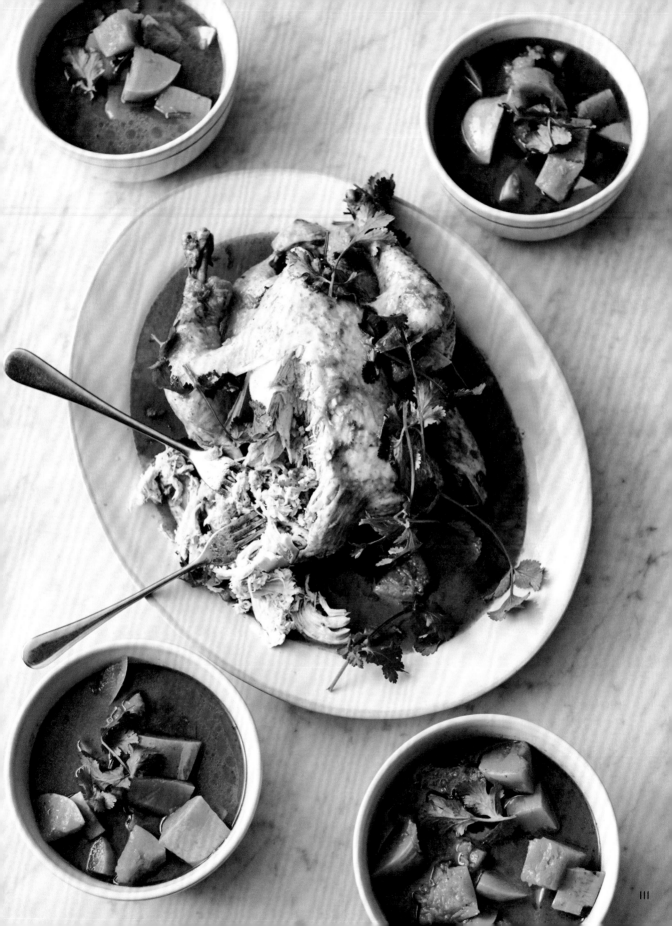

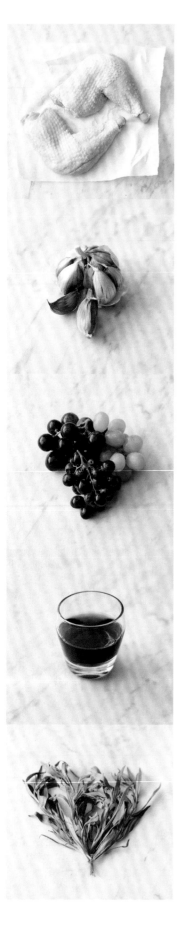

SWEET CHICKEN SURPRISE

SERVES 2   FAST PREP 8 MINUTES   COOK 40 MINUTES

2 x 200g chicken legs

1 bulb of garlic

250g mixed-colour seedless grapes

100ml red vermouth

4 sprigs of fresh tarragon

Preheat the oven to 180°C/350°F/gas 4. Put a non-stick ovenproof frying pan on a high heat. Rub the chicken all over with ½ a tablespoon of olive oil, season with sea salt and black pepper and place skin side down in the pan. Fry for a couple of minutes until golden, then lightly squash the unpeeled garlic cloves with the heel of your hand and add to the pan. Pick in the grapes.

Turn the chicken skin side up, pour in the vermouth and transfer to the oven to roast for 40 minutes, or until the chicken is golden and tender, and the sauce is sticky and reduced. Add a splash of water to the pan and give it a gentle shimmy to pick up all the sticky bits. Pick over the tarragon, and dish up.

CALORIES	FAT	SAT FAT	PROTEIN	CARBS	SUGAR	SALT	FIBRE
440kcal	22.2g	5.6g	28g	25.8g	22g	0.8g	1.6g

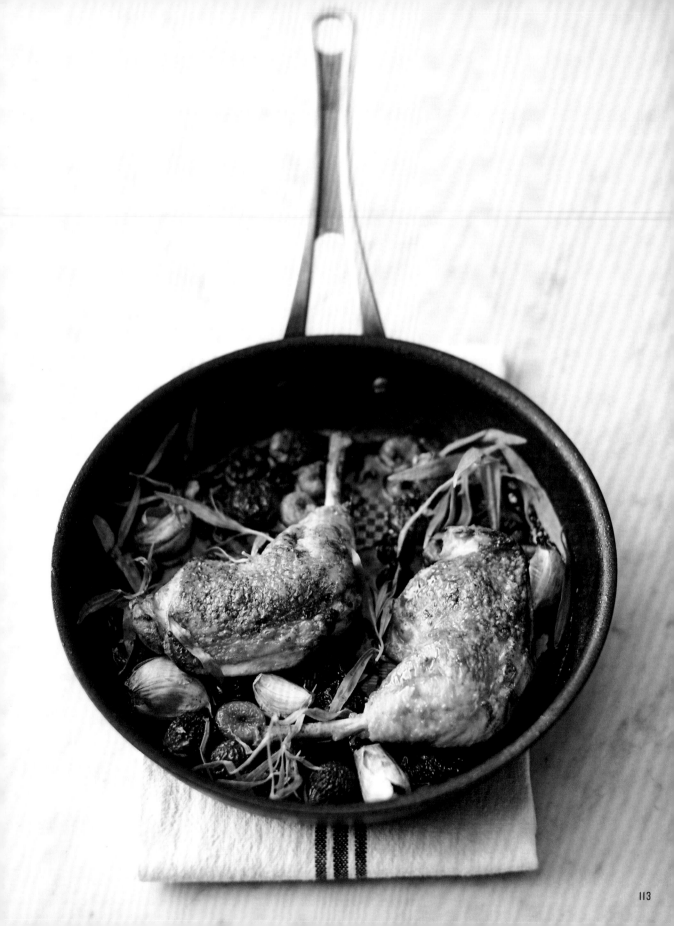

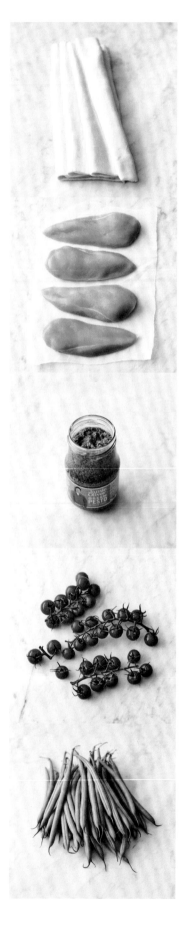

FLAKY PASTRY PESTO CHICKEN

SERVES 4   TOTAL 30 MINUTES

320g sheet of all-butter puff pastry (cold)

4 x 120g skinless chicken breasts

4 heaped teaspoons green pesto

400g ripe cherry tomatoes, on the vine

400g green beans

Preheat the oven to 220°C/425°F/gas 7. Unroll the pastry, cut it in half lengthways, then cut each half widthways into 8 equal strips. Flatten the chicken breasts by pounding with your fist until the fat ends are the same thickness as the skinny ends. Place them in a roasting tray, season with sea salt and black pepper, spread over the pesto, then lay 4 overlapping strips of pastry over each breast, tucking them under at the edges. Brush with a little olive oil. Lightly dress the tomato vines in olive oil, season and put into a second tray. Place the chicken tray on the top shelf of the oven with the tomatoes below, and cook for 20 minutes, or until the pastry is golden and the chicken is cooked through.

Meanwhile, line up the beans, trim off just the stalk ends, then cook in a pan of boiling salted water for 7 minutes, or until tender. Remove the chicken to a board with half the tomatoes, squashing the rest in the tray and discarding the vines. Drain and toss in the beans, taste and season to perfection. Slice the chicken at an angle and serve on top of the beans, with the whole tomatoes.

CALORIES	FAT	SAT FAT	PROTEIN	CARBS	SUGAR	SALT	FIBRE
618kcal	34.8g	18g	36.3g	40.4g	7.1g	1.7g	4.9g

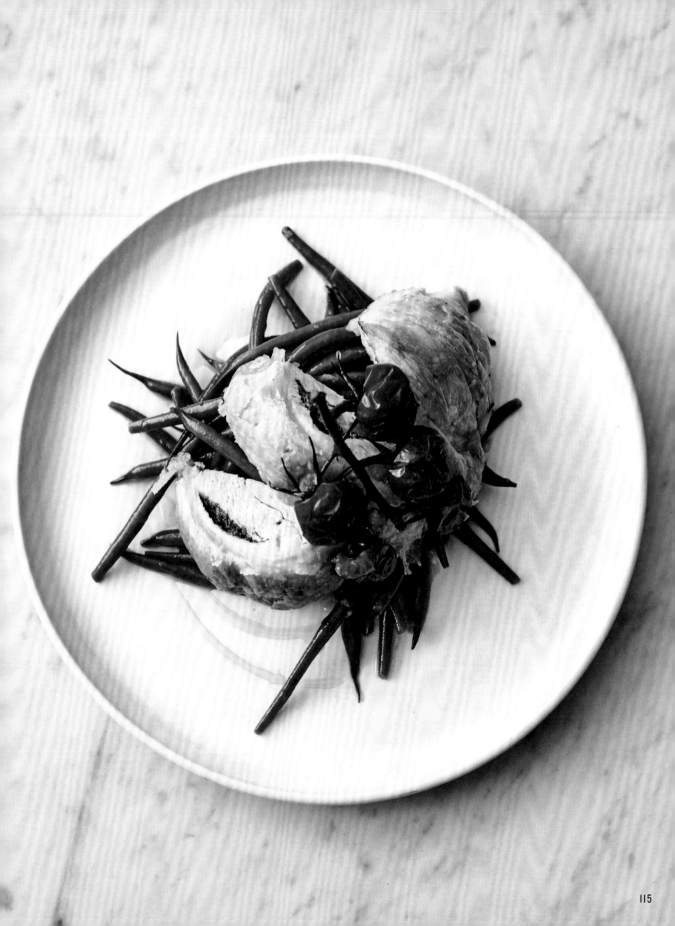

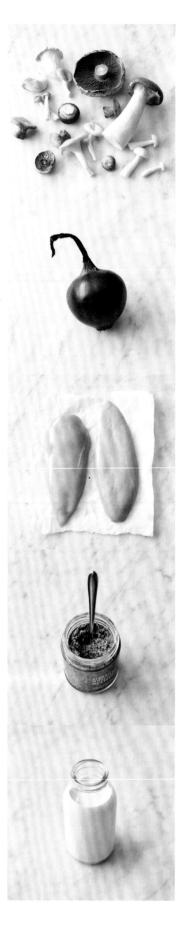

CREAMY MUSTARD CHICKEN

SERVES 2   TOTAL 20 MINUTES

200g mixed mushrooms

1 red onion

2 x 120g skinless chicken breasts

2 teaspoons wholegrain mustard

60ml single cream

Place a 30cm non-stick frying pan on a medium-high heat. Place all the mushrooms in the dry pan, tearing up any larger ones. Let them toast and get dark golden and nutty, tossing occasionally, while you peel and finely slice the red onion and slice the chicken breasts into 1cm-thick strips.

When the mushrooms look good, add the onion and chicken to the pan with 1 tablespoon of olive oil. Cook for 5 minutes, tossing often, then add the mustard, cream and 150ml of water. Bring to the boil, then simmer until you've just got a loose saucy consistency and the chicken is cooked through. Taste, season to perfection with sea salt and black pepper, and dish up.

CALORIES	FAT	SAT FAT	PROTEIN	CARBS	SUGAR	SALT	FIBRE
304kcal	16.1g	5.4g	32.8g	7.6g	5.6g	0.5g	2.5g

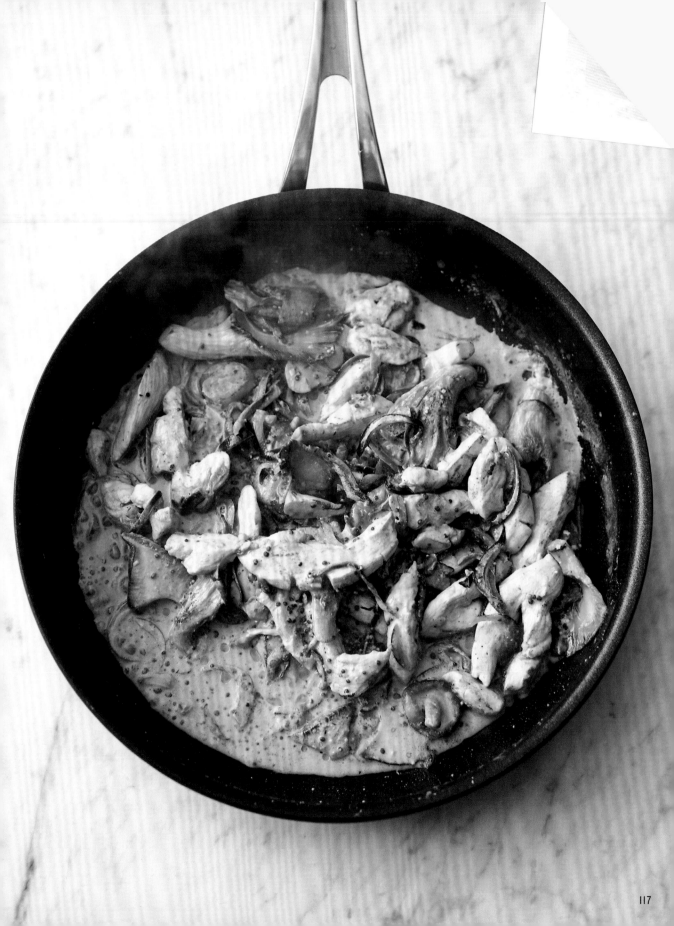

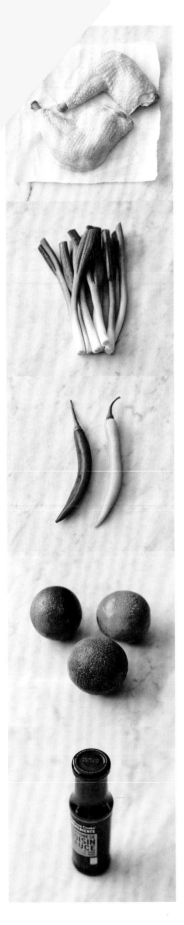

STICKY HOISIN CHICKEN

SERVES 2 | TOTAL 30 MINUTES

2 x 200g chicken legs

8 spring onions

1–2 fresh mixed-colour chillies

3 regular or blood oranges

2 heaped tablespoons hoisin sauce

Preheat the oven to 180°C/350°F/gas 4. Put a non-stick ovenproof frying pan on a high heat. Pull off the chicken skin, put both skin and legs into the pan, season with sea salt and black pepper and let the fat render out and the chicken get golden for 5 minutes, turning halfway, while you trim the spring onions and halve across the middle, putting the green halves aside. Toss the white spring onions into the pan, then transfer to the oven for 15 minutes. Meanwhile, deseed the chillies, then finely slice lengthways with the green spring onions and pop both into a bowl of ice-cold water to curl and crisp up. Peel the oranges, finely slice into rounds, and arrange on your plates.

Remove the chicken skin and soft spring onions from the pan and put aside. Cook the chicken for 10 more minutes, or until tender and cooked through. In a bowl, loosen the hoisin with a splash of red wine vinegar, then spoon over the chicken. Leave it in the oven while you drain and divide up the salad. Sit the chicken and soft spring onions on top and crack over the crispy skin.

CALORIES	FAT	SAT FAT	PROTEIN	CARBS	SUGAR	SALT	FIBRE
430kcal	19.5g	5.2g	29g	36.2g	35g	1.5g	4g

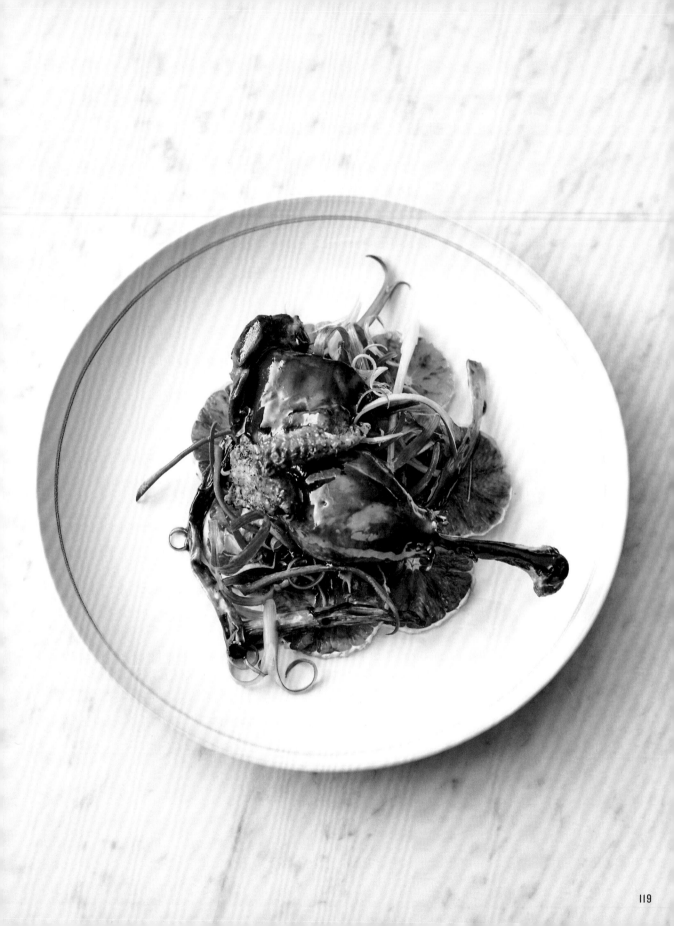

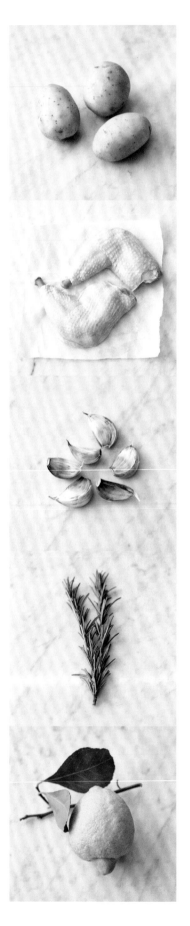

HERBY CHICKEN TRAYBAKE

SERVES 2   FAST PREP 8 MINUTES   COOK 50 MINUTES

400g potatoes

2 x 200g chicken legs

6 cloves of garlic

2 sprigs of fresh rosemary

1 lemon

Preheat the oven to 180°C/350°F/gas 4. Scrub the potatoes, slice just under ½cm thick, and place in a 25cm x 30cm roasting tray with the chicken, ½ a tablespoon of olive oil and a pinch of sea salt and black pepper. Lightly squash and add the unpeeled garlic cloves, toss well, then arrange the spuds in a fairly even layer. Sit the chicken legs directly on the bars of the oven, skin side up, with the tray of potatoes directly underneath. Bake for 40 minutes.

When the time's up, mix up the potatoes in the tasty tray juices, then sit the chicken on top. Strip the rosemary leaves off the sprigs, use a speed-peeler to peel strips of lemon zest, then toss both in 1 teaspoon of olive oil and sprinkle into the tray. Squeeze over half the lemon juice, then return to the oven for a final 10 minutes, or until the chicken is tender and super-golden.

CALORIES	FAT	SAT FAT	PROTEIN	CARBS	SUGAR	SALT	FIBRE
490kcal	25.4g	6g	30.4g	37.2g	1.4g	0.8g	3.2g

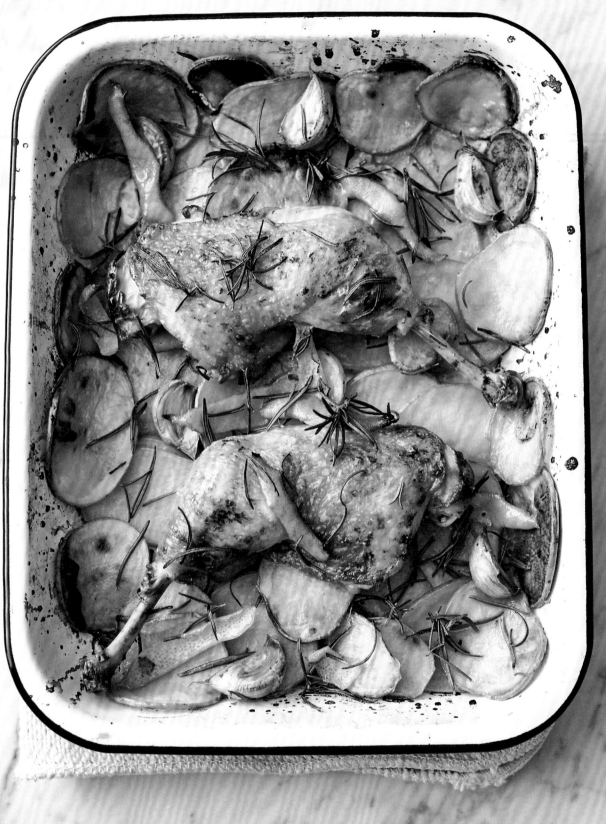

FISH

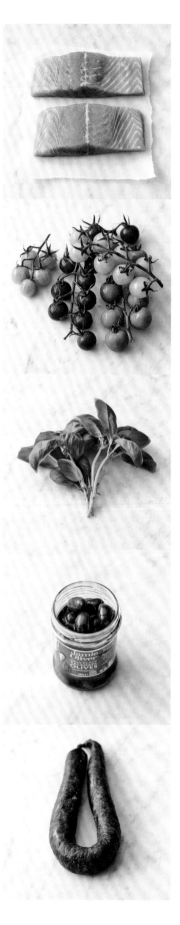

SMOKY CHORIZO SALMON

SERVES 2   TOTAL JUST 11 MINUTES

2 x 150g salmon fillets, skin on, scaled, pin-boned

300g ripe mixed-colour cherry tomatoes

4 sprigs of fresh basil

8 black olives (stone in)

30g chorizo

Put the salmon flesh side down in a large cold non-stick frying pan and place on a medium-high heat. As the pan comes up to temperature and the salmon begins to sizzle (about 3 minutes), flip it over and cook on the skin side for 5 minutes, or until very crisp and just cooked (depending on its thickness).

Meanwhile, halve the cherry tomatoes, tear up most of the basil leaves, then toss it all with 1 tablespoon of red wine vinegar and a pinch of sea salt and black pepper. Squash the olives and discard the stones, then finely chop the flesh. Mix with 1 teaspoon of extra virgin olive oil and a splash of water.

Finely slice the chorizo, add to the pan for the last 2 minutes, then toss in the dressed tomatoes for 30 seconds. Divide between your plates, with the salmon on top. Spoon over the dressed olives and pick over the remaining basil.

CALORIES	FAT	SAT FAT	PROTEIN	CARBS	SUGAR	SALT	FIBRE
363kcal	22.8g	4.8g	34.3g	5.1g	4.9g	1.2g	1.5g

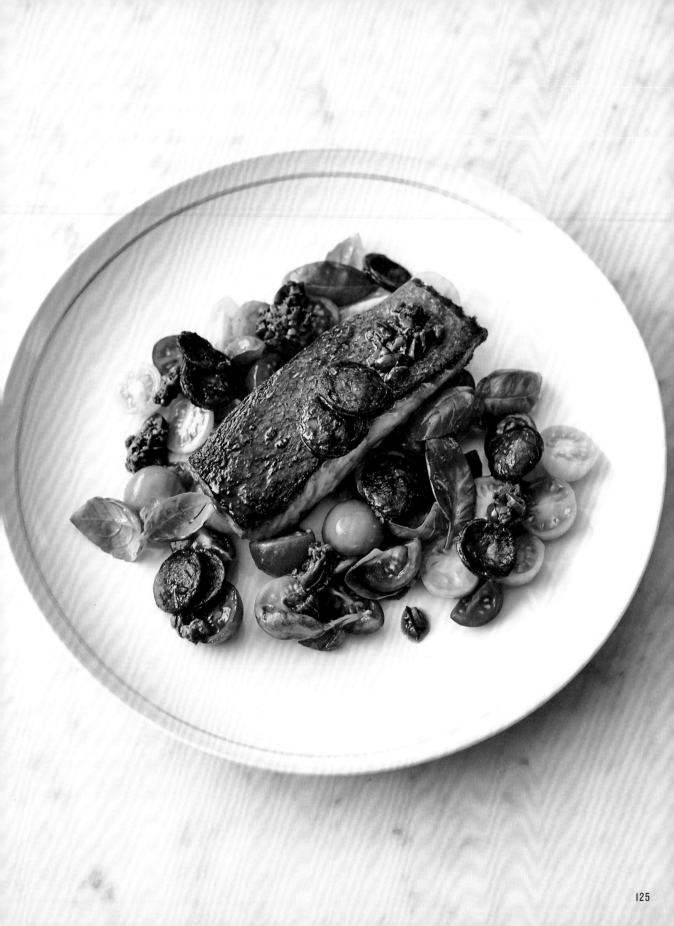

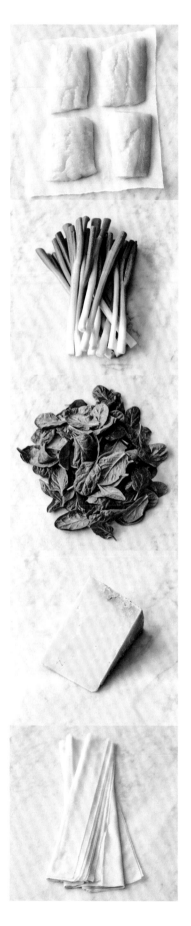

CRAZY SIMPLE FISH PIE

SERVES 4   TOTAL 28 MINUTES

400g undyed smoked haddock, skin off

2 bunches of spring onions

250g baby spinach

150g Cheddar cheese

4 sheets of filo pastry

Preheat the oven to 200°C/400°F/gas 6. In a bowl, cover the fish with boiling kettle water. Put aside to soak while you trim and roughly chop the spring onions, placing them into a 30cm non-stick ovenproof frying pan on a high heat with 1 tablespoon of olive oil. Stir and fry for 2 minutes, then pile the spinach on top, let it wilt down and turn the heat off.

Spoon 100ml of the soaking water over the spinach, then drain the fish, break up the pieces and sit them evenly around the pan. Finely grate over most of the cheese and season well with black pepper. Quickly layer the filo on top, tucking it around the fish and up the sides of the pan, tearing the last sheet on top in a nutty fashion. Grate over the last bit of cheese, drizzle with ½ a tablespoon of olive oil, and bake for 15 to 17 minutes, or until golden and crisp. Easy as pie!

CALORIES	FAT	SAT FAT	PROTEIN	CARBS	SUGAR	SALT	FIBRE
431kcal	20.9g	9.3g	34.5g	27.9g	3.4g	3.2g	3.5g

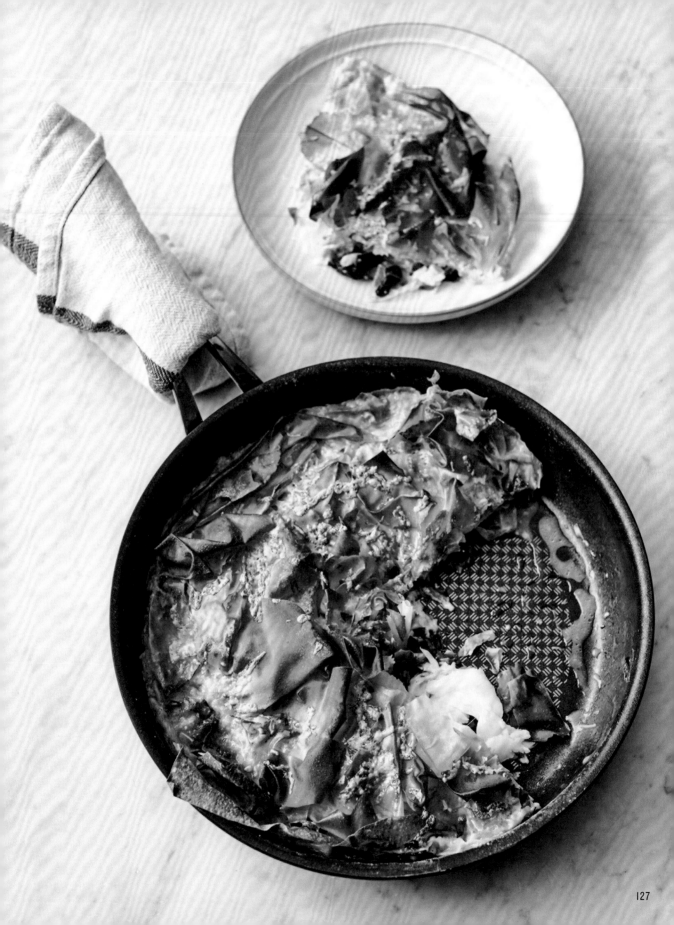

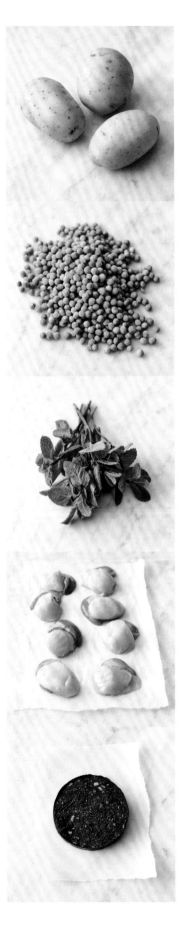

SIZZLING SEARED SCALLOPS

SERVES 2   TOTAL 18 MINUTES

400g potatoes

200g frozen peas

½ a bunch of fresh mint (15g)

6–8 raw king scallops, coral attached, trimmed

50g firm black pudding

Wash the potatoes, chop into 3cm chunks and cook in a pan of boiling salted water for 12 minutes, or until tender, adding the peas for the last 3 minutes. Meanwhile, pick and finely chop most of the mint leaves and put aside. Place a non-stick frying pan on a medium-high heat. Once hot, put 1 tablespoon of olive oil and the remaining mint leaves in to crisp up for 1 minute, then scoop the leaves on to a plate, leaving the oil behind. Season the scallops with sea salt and black pepper and fry for 2 minutes on each side, or until golden. Crumble in the black pudding (discarding the skin) so it crisps up alongside.

Drain the peas and potatoes, return to the pan, mash well with the chopped mint and 1 tablespoon of extra virgin olive oil, taste and season to perfection. Plate up with the scallops and black pudding, drizzle lightly with extra virgin olive oil, and sprinkle over the crispy mint.

CALORIES	FAT	SAT FAT	PROTEIN	CARBS	SUGAR	SALT	FIBRE
517kcal	23.6g	5g	27.4g	52g	3.6g	1.3g	7.9g

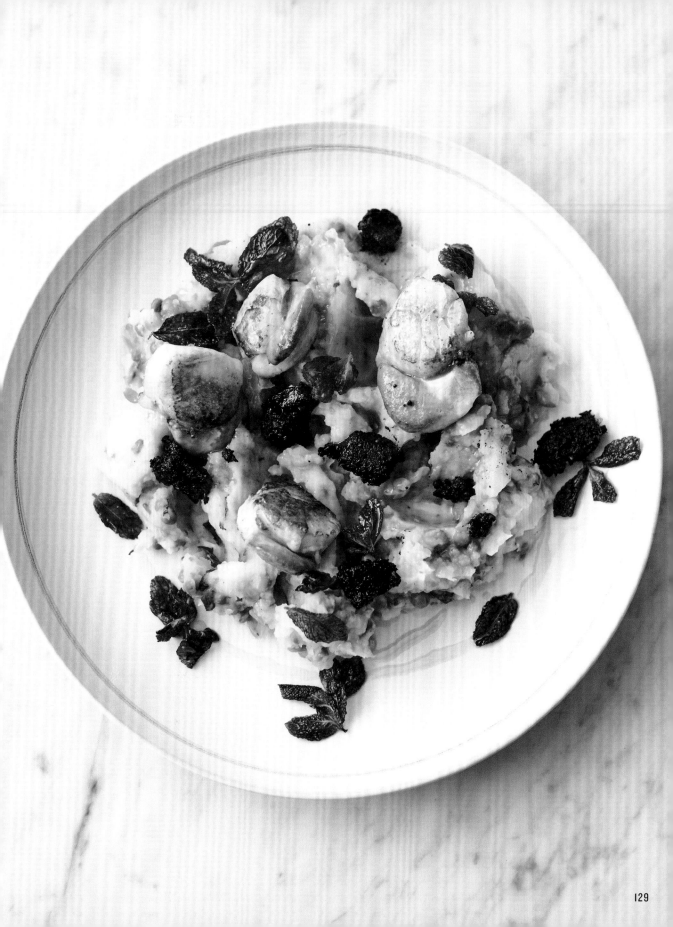

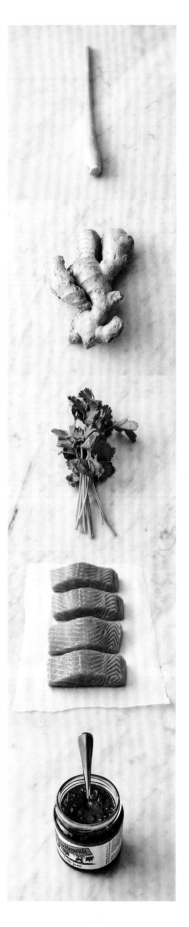

QUICK ASIAN FISHCAKES

MAKES 4 | TOTAL 22 MINUTES

1 stick of lemongrass

6cm piece of ginger

½ a bunch of fresh coriander (15g)

500g salmon fillets, skin off, pin-boned

4 teaspoons chilli jam

Whack the lemongrass against your work surface and remove the tough outer layer. Peel the ginger, then very finely chop with the inside of the lemongrass and most of the coriander, stalks and all, reserving a few nice leaves in a bowl of cold water. Chop the salmon into 1cm chunks over the mix on your board, then push half the salmon to one side. Chop the rest until super-fine, almost like a purée, then mix the chunkier bits back through it and season with sea salt and black pepper. Divide into 4, then shape and squash into 2cm-thick patties.

Place a large non-stick frying pan on a medium-high heat with 1 tablespoon of olive oil. Cook the patties for 2 minutes on each side, or until nicely golden. Spoon the chilli jam over the fishcakes, add a splash of water to the pan, turn the heat off, and jiggle to coat. Serve sprinkled with the drained coriander.

CALORIES	FAT	SAT FAT	PROTEIN	CARBS	SUGAR	SALT	FIBRE
277kcal	17.2g	2.9g	25.7g	4.8g	3.8g	0.7g	0.1g

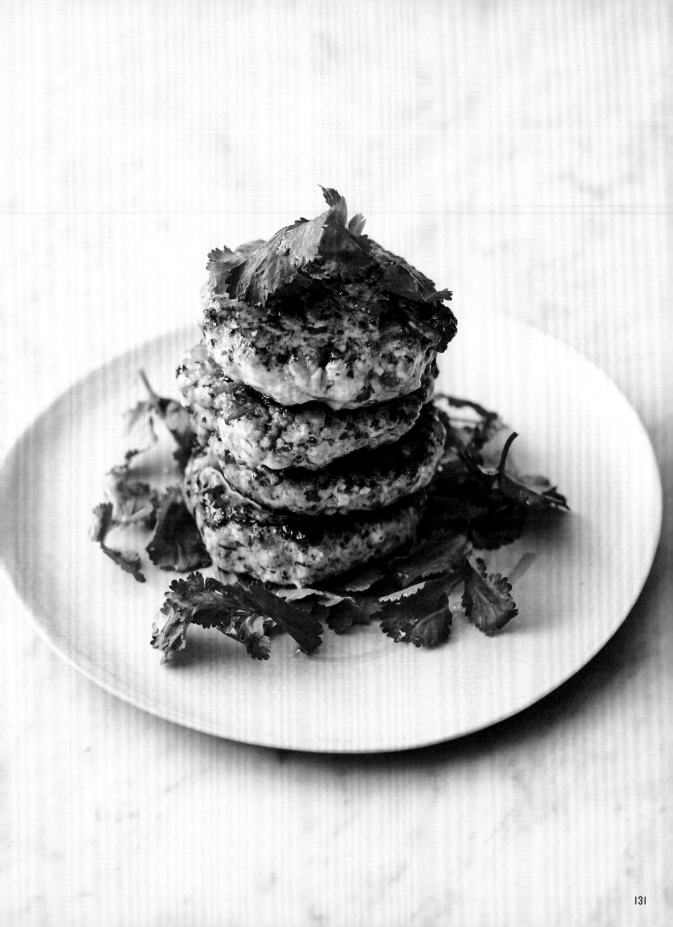

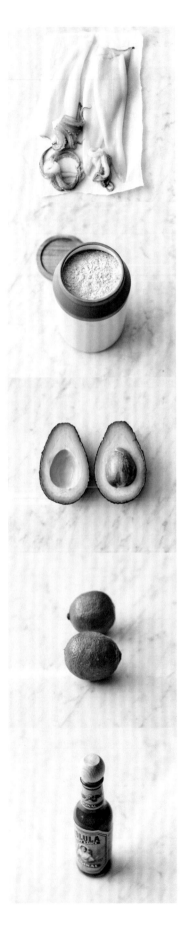

CRISPY SQUID & SMASHED AVO

SERVES 2   TOTAL 20 MINUTES

250g squid, gutted, cleaned

2 heaped tablespoons wholemeal flour

1 ripe avocado

2 limes

2 teaspoons hot chilli sauce

Pour 1cm of olive oil into a large non-stick frying pan on a medium-high heat and leave to get hot – keep an eye on it. Meanwhile, slice the squid tubes into 1cm rings, then toss all the squid with the flour and a pinch of sea salt and black pepper until well coated. Halve and destone the avocado, then scoop the flesh into a bowl. Finely grate in the zest of 1 lime, squeeze in the juice, and mash until smooth. Taste, season to perfection, and divide between two plates.

To test if the oil is hot enough, carefully drop a piece of squid into the pan – if it sizzles and turns golden, it's ready. Piece by piece, gently place the rest of the squid in the hot oil and cook, turning with tongs, until golden all over (work in batches, if you need to). Remove to a plate lined with kitchen paper to drain, then plate up over the avo. Drizzle over the chilli sauce and a little extra virgin olive oil, and serve with lime wedges, for squeezing over.

CALORIES	FAT	SAT FAT	PROTEIN	CARBS	SUGAR	SALT	FIBRE
473kcal	29.3g	5g	25.4g	28.7g	1.8g	1g	3.7g

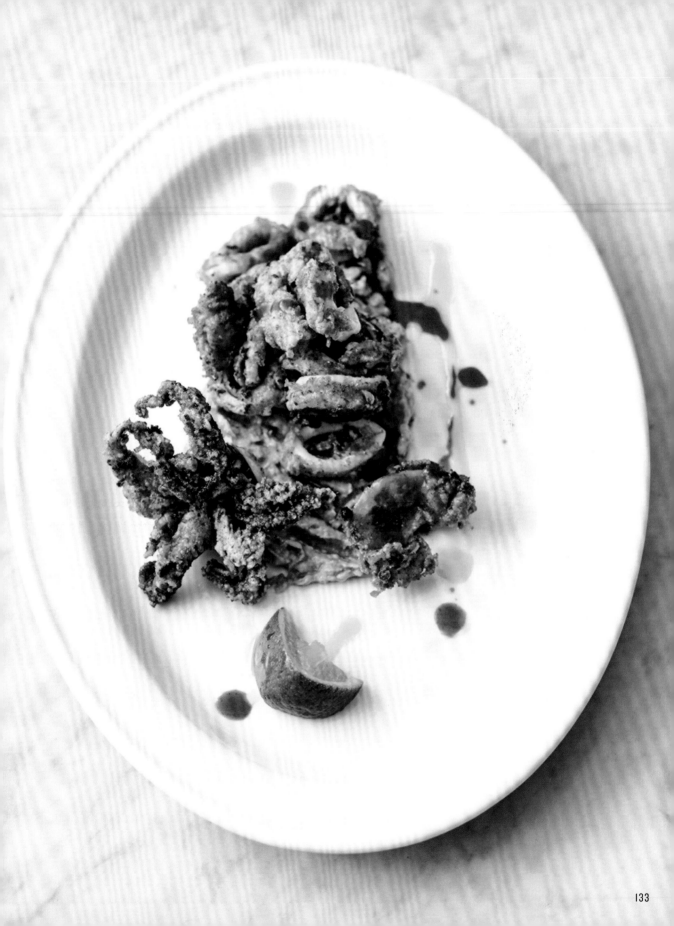

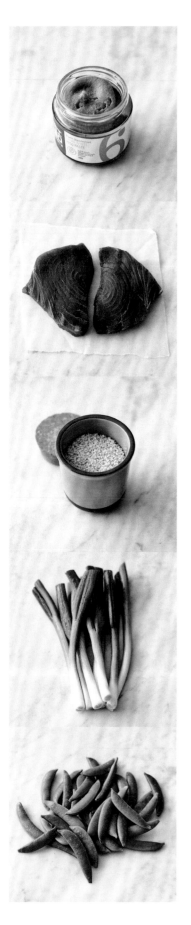

SEARED SESAME TUNA

SERVES 2 | TOTAL JUST 10 MINUTES

1 heaped tablespoon miso paste

2 x 150g tuna steaks (ideally 2cm thick)

4 tablespoons sesame seeds

8 spring onions

150g sugar snap peas

Place a large non-stick frying pan on a medium-high heat. Rub the miso all over the tuna, then pat on the sesame seeds to cover. Place in the hot pan with 1 tablespoon of olive oil and sear for 1½ minutes on each side, so it's beautifully golden on the outside but blushing in the middle. Remove to a board to rest. Quickly wipe out the pan with a ball of kitchen paper, then return to the heat.

Trim the spring onions and slice at an angle the same length as the sugar snaps, tossing both into the hot pan with a few drips of red wine vinegar and a pinch of sea salt for 2 minutes to lightly catch and char. Slice the sesame tuna and serve on top of the veg, drizzled with 1 teaspoon of extra virgin olive oil.

CALORIES	FAT	SAT FAT	PROTEIN	CARBS	SUGAR	SALT	FIBRE
450kcal	27.4g	5.1g	43.9g	7.5g	4g	1.1g	3.3g

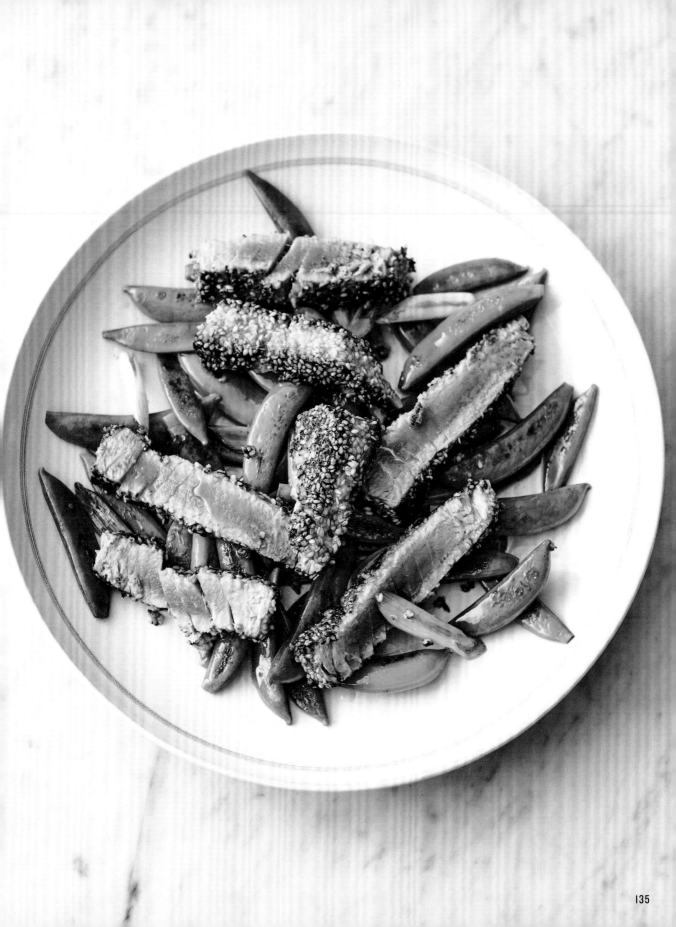

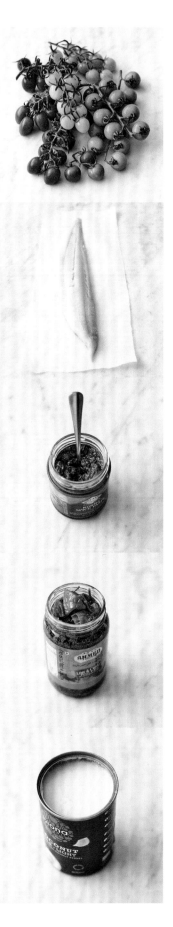

SO EASY FISH CURRY

SERVES 4 | TOTAL JUST 14 MINUTES

500g ripe mixed-colour cherry tomatoes

500g white fish fillets, such as haddock, skin off, pin-boned

1 heaped tablespoon korma curry paste

1 tablespoon lime pickle

1 x 400ml tin of light coconut milk

Place 1 tablespoon of olive oil in a large shallow casserole pan on a high heat. Halve the tomatoes, adding them to the pan skin side down. Blister for 2 minutes without moving them while you chop the haddock into 4cm chunks.

Stir the haddock, korma paste, lime pickle and coconut milk into the pan. Bring to the boil, then simmer for 6 minutes, taking care not to break up the fish. Taste, season to perfection with sea salt and black pepper, then dish up. Joy.

CALORIES	FAT	SAT FAT	PROTEIN	CARBS	SUGAR	SALT	FIBRE
257kcal	13.3g	6g	26.4g	8.2g	7g	0.9g	2.1g

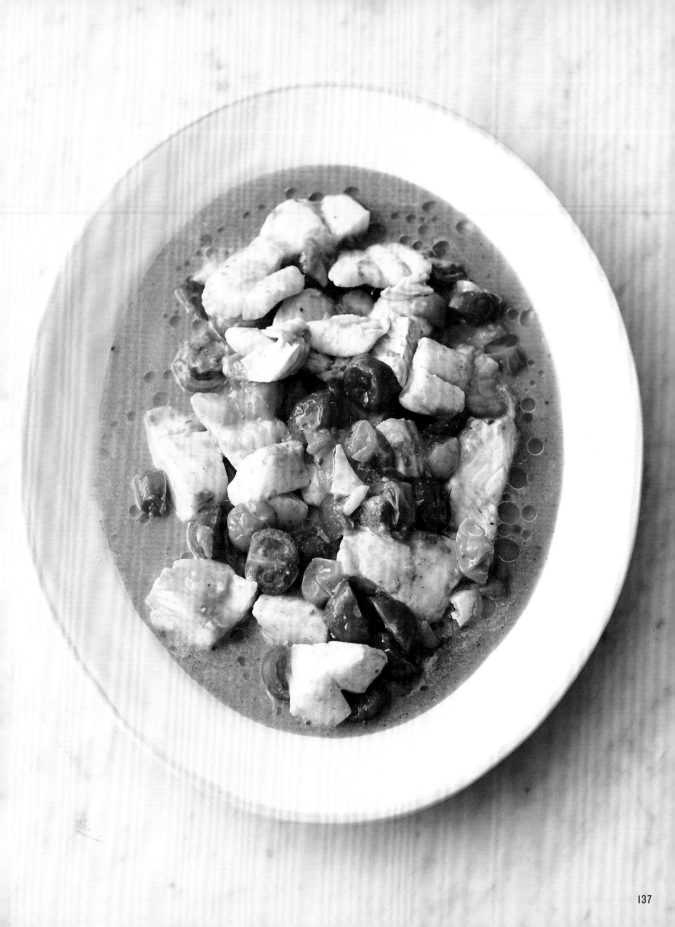

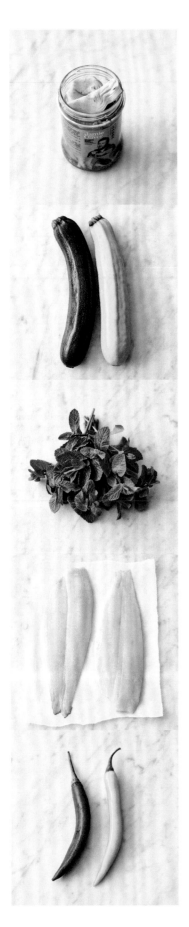

CRISPY SKIN LEMON SOLE

SERVES 2   TOTAL 20 MINUTES

½ x 280g jar of artichoke hearts in oil

2 mixed-colour courgettes

1 bunch of fresh mint (30g)

2 x 200g sides of flat white fish, such as lemon sole, skin on, scaled

1–2 fresh mixed-colour chillies

Preheat the grill to high. Scoop out the artichokes, halve lengthways and place in a large non-stick ovenproof frying pan on a medium heat with 1 tablespoon of oil from their jar. Quarter the courgettes lengthways, cut out the core, slice them at an angle the same size as the artichokes and add to the pan. Cook for 10 minutes, stirring regularly. Finely slice the top leafy half of the mint, tossing half into the pan with a splash of water.

Rub the sole with a little olive oil, sea salt and black pepper, then lay skin side up on the veg. Place the pan directly under the grill for 7 to 10 minutes, or until the skin is wonderfully crisp – keep an eye on it! Meanwhile, finely slice the chillies, mix as much as you dare with the remaining mint, 2 tablespoons of red wine vinegar and 1 tablespoon of extra virgin olive oil, then taste and season to perfection. Plate up the veg and sole, pulling back half the crispy skin to expose the fish, then drizzle over the chilli mint dressing.

CALORIES	FAT	SAT FAT	PROTEIN	CARBS	SUGAR	SALT	FIBRE
309kcal	13.6g	2g	38.8g	5.9g	3.7g	2.8g	3.3g

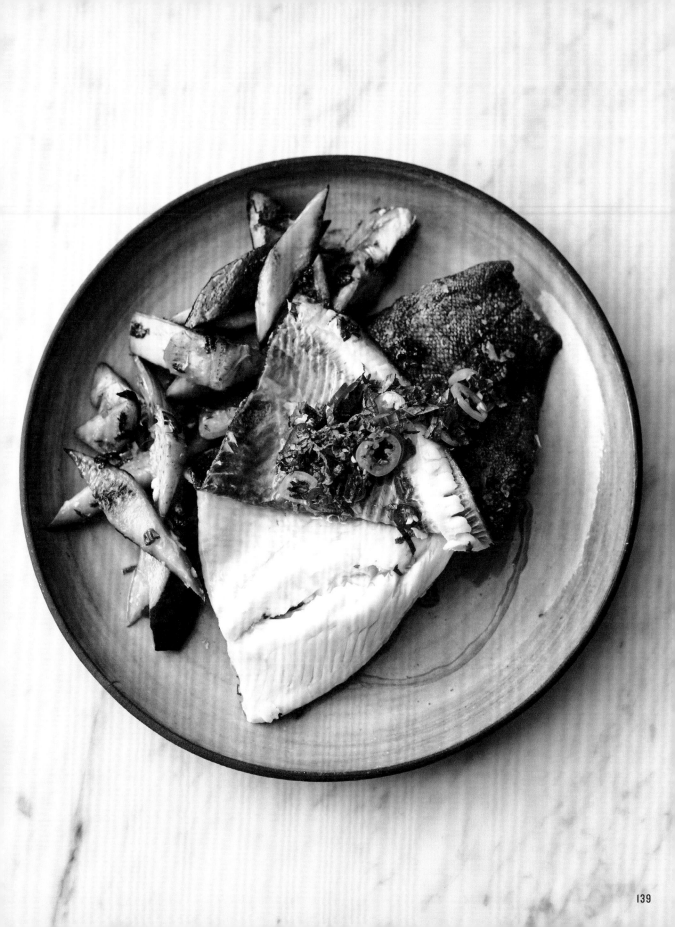

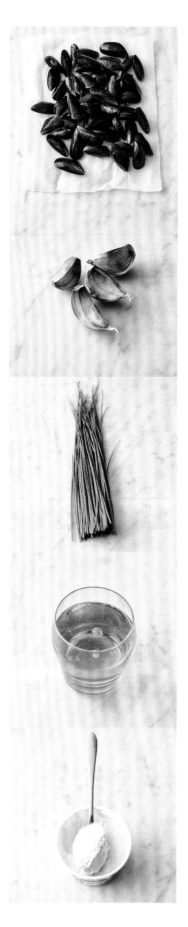

CREAMY CORNISH MUSSELS

SERVES 2 | TOTAL JUST 12 MINUTES

600g mussels, scrubbed, debearded

4 cloves of garlic

1 bunch of fresh chives (30g)

250ml Cornish cider

50g clotted cream

Check the mussels – if any are open, give them a tap and they should close; if they don't, discard them. Peel and finely slice the garlic. Finely chop the chives.

Put a large deep pan on a high heat. Pour in 1 tablespoon of olive oil, then add the garlic and most of the chives, followed 1 minute later by the cider. Bring to a fast boil, then add the mussels and clotted cream, cover and leave for 3 to 4 minutes, shaking the pan occasionally. When all the mussels have opened and are soft and juicy, they're ready. If any remain closed, discard them.

Taste the sauce, season to perfection with sea salt and black pepper, then dish up and sprinkle over the remaining chives before tucking in.

CALORIES	FAT	SAT FAT	PROTEIN	CARBS	SUGAR	SALT	FIBRE
347kcal	24.6g	11.2g	15.2g	8.4g	4.2g	0.8g	0.7g

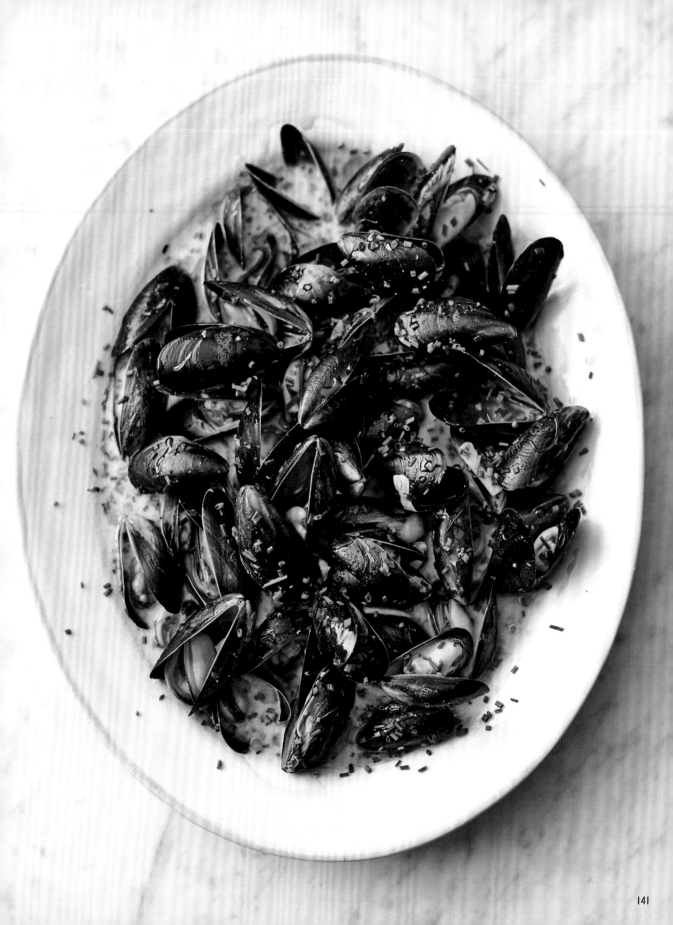

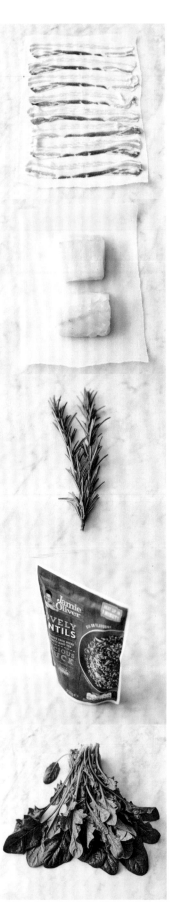

SMOKY PANCETTA COD

SERVES 2 | TOTAL 16 MINUTES

8 rashers of smoked pancetta

2 x 150g white fish fillets, such as cod, skin off, pin-boned

2 sprigs of fresh rosemary

1 x 250g sachet of cooked lentils

200g spinach

Lay out 4 rashers of pancetta, slightly overlapping them. Place a piece of cod on top, generously season with black pepper, then roll and wrap in the pancetta, and repeat. Place in a large non-stick frying pan on a medium heat and cook for 8 minutes, turning occasionally, adding the rosemary for the last 2 minutes.

Remove the fish to a plate. Toss the lentils into the pan with 1 tablespoon of red wine vinegar and push to one side to reheat for 1 minute and pick up all that residual flavour, while you quickly wilt the spinach with a splash of water alongside. Taste, season to perfection with sea salt and pepper, and divide both between your plates. Sit the wrapped cod on top of the lentils with the rosemary, and drizzle with 1 teaspoon of extra virgin olive oil.

CALORIES	FAT	SAT FAT	PROTEIN	CARBS	SUGAR	SALT	FIBRE
348kcal	9.2g	2.4g	44.1g	22.9g	2g	1.2g	2.1g

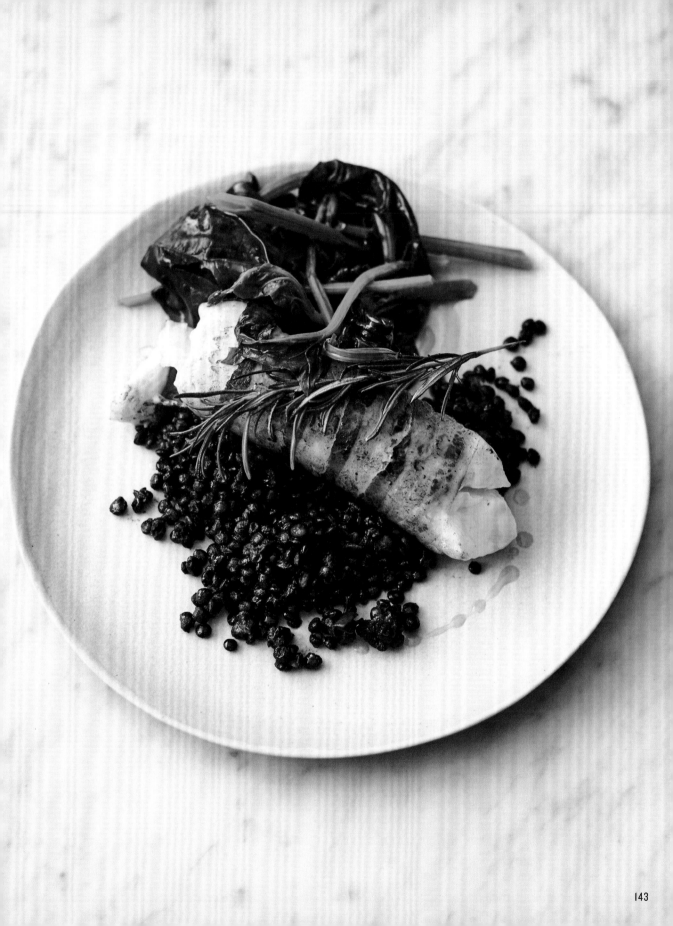

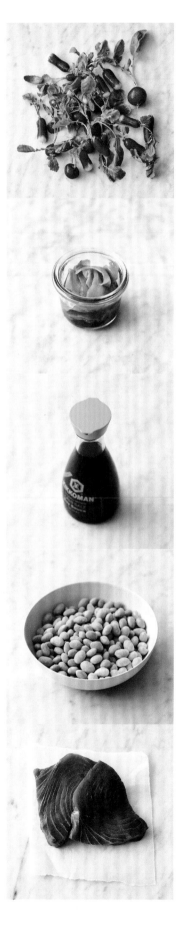

ASIAN TUNA STEAK SALAD

SERVES 2   TOTAL JUST 10 MINUTES

200g radishes, ideally with leaves

2 heaped teaspoons pickled ginger

2 teaspoons low-salt soy sauce

250g frozen soya beans

2 x 150g tuna steaks (ideally 2cm thick)

Finely chop 2 radishes with the pickled ginger, then dress with the soy, 1 tablespoon of extra virgin olive oil and 2 teaspoons of water and put aside. Very finely slice the remaining radishes with their leaves.

Place the beans in a non-stick frying pan on a high heat, cover with boiling kettle water, boil for 2 minutes, then drain. Return the pan to a medium-high heat. Rub the tuna with 1 teaspoon of olive oil and a pinch of sea salt and black pepper, then sear for 1½ minutes on each side, so it's blushing in the middle.

Divide the beans and radishes between your plates, half-tear the tuna and place proudly on top, then spoon over the pickled ginger mixture, drizzling all the juices around the plate. Finish with 1 teaspoon of extra virgin olive oil.

CALORIES	FAT	SAT FAT	PROTEIN	CARBS	SUGAR	SALT	FIBRE
426kcal	19.2g	3.5g	54g	9.8g	5g	1.3g	0.1g

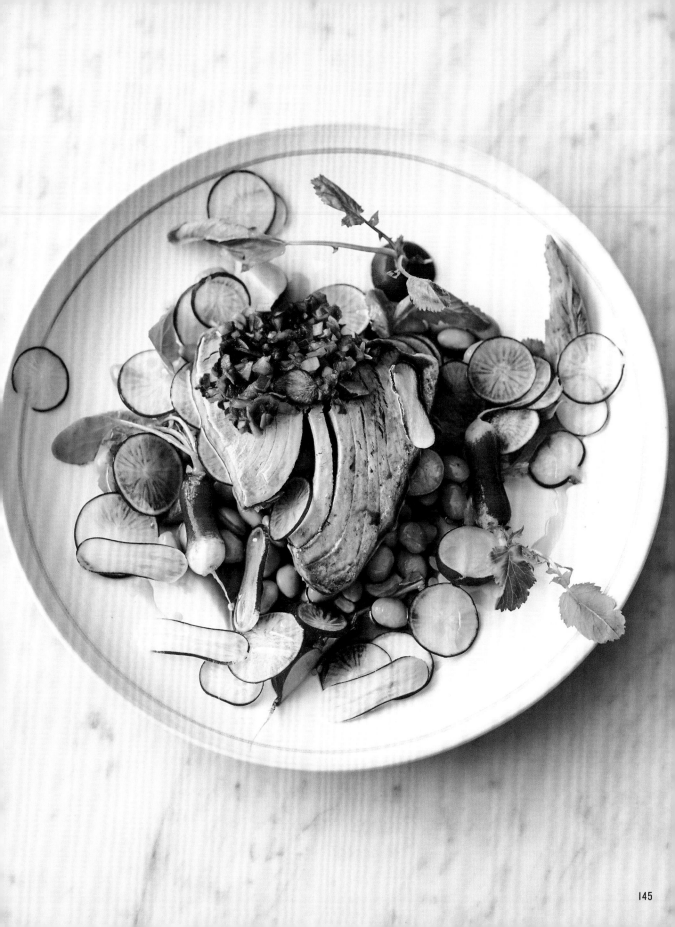

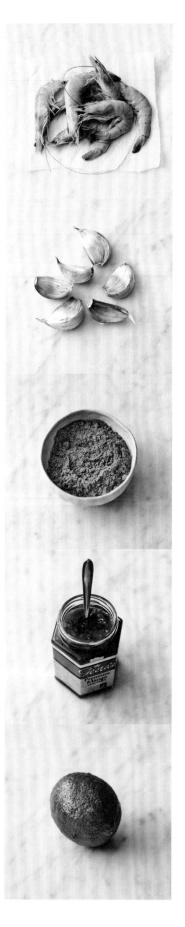

STICKY MANGO PRAWNS

SERVES 2   TOTAL 20 MINUTES

300g large raw shell-on king prawns

6 cloves of garlic

1 teaspoon curry powder

1 heaped tablespoon mango chutney

1 lime

Quickly pull the legs and tails off the prawns and peel off the shells, leaving the heads on for bonus flavour. Run the tip of your knife down their backs and pull out the vein. Put a large non-stick frying pan on a medium heat. Peel and very finely slice the garlic, fry with 1 tablespoon of olive oil until crisp, then scoop out and put aside, leaving the garlicky oil behind.

Stir the curry powder into the oil, then add the prawns. Fry for 4 minutes, or until the prawns are cooked through, tossing regularly. Stir in the mango chutney for 30 seconds, taste, season to perfection with sea salt and black pepper, then dish up. Scatter over the crispy garlic, finely grate over half the lime zest and serve with lime wedges, for squeezing over.

CALORIES	FAT	SAT FAT	PROTEIN	CARBS	SUGAR	SALT	FIBRE
168kcal	7.3g	1.1g	15.8g	10.4g	7.4g	0.9g	0.9g

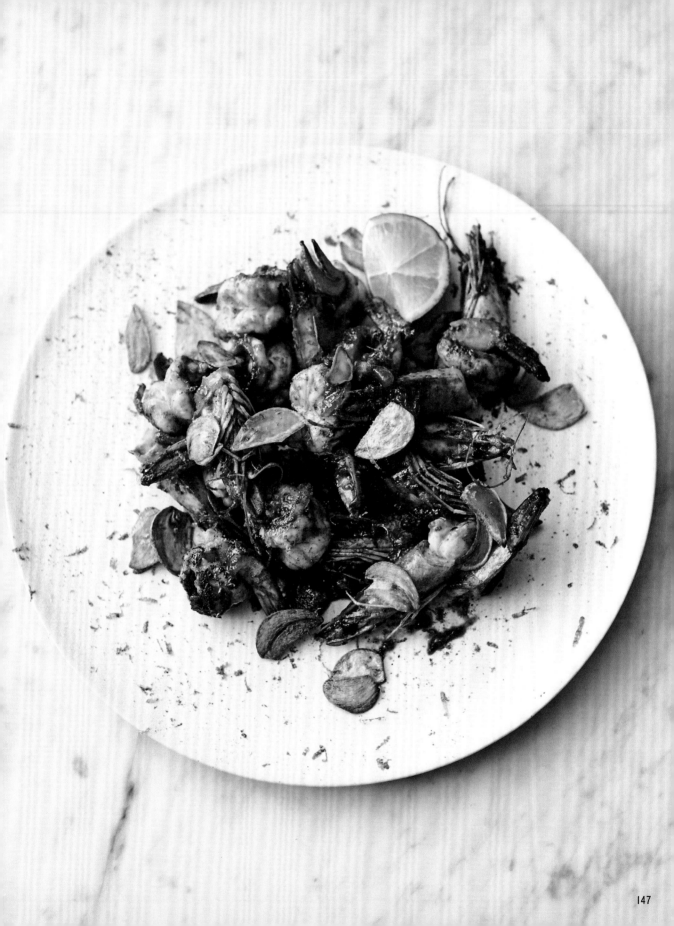

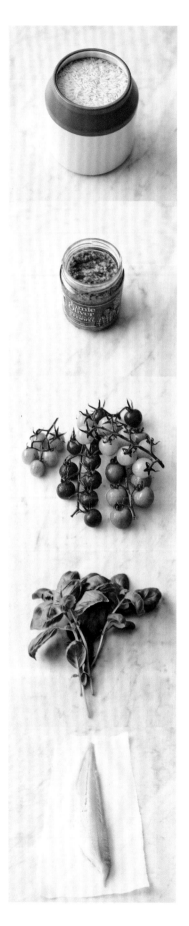

ONE-PAN FABULOUS FISH

SERVES 4   TOTAL JUST 15 MINUTES

300g white basmati rice

6 heaped teaspoons green olive tapenade

350g ripe mixed-colour cherry tomatoes

½ a bunch of fresh basil (15g)

500g white fish fillets, such as haddock, skin off, pin-boned

In a large shallow casserole pan on a high heat, mix the rice with 2 heaped teaspoons of tapenade, then pour over 600ml of water. Put the lid on and let it come to the boil while you halve the tomatoes and, in a bowl, mix them with 1 tablespoon each of olive oil and red wine vinegar. Taste, season to perfection with sea salt and black pepper, and tear in most of the basil leaves.

Cut the fish into four equal-sized pieces and place in the pan, pushing them into the rice. Scatter over the dressed tomatoes. Put the lid back on and boil for 10 minutes, or until the rice is cooked through, then remove the lid and cook for a further 2 minutes until all the liquid has evaporated. Spoon the remaining tapenade over the fish, pick over the remaining basil leaves, drizzle lightly with extra virgin olive oil, and dish up.

CALORIES	FAT	SAT FAT	PROTEIN	CARBS	SUGAR	SALT	FIBRE
484kcal	12g	1.7g	31.2g	66.7g	3.8g	1.2g	2.7g

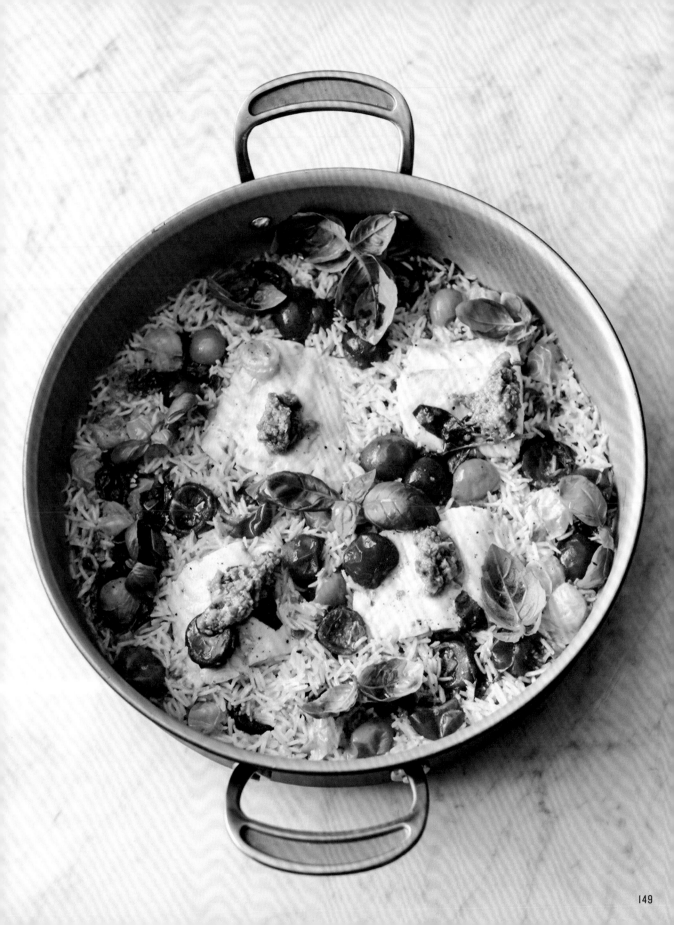

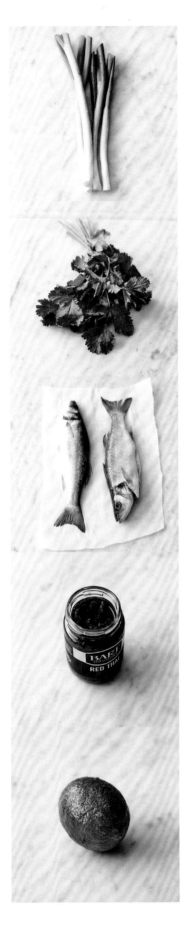

THAI-STYLE CRISPY SEA BASS

SERVES 2 | TOTAL 19 MINUTES

4 spring onions

½ a bunch of fresh coriander (15g)

2 x 300g whole sea bass, scaled, gutted, trimmed

2 tablespoons Thai red curry paste

1 lime

Trim and halve the spring onions, finely shred lengthways and place in a bowl of ice-cold water to crisp up. Pick in the coriander leaves, reserving the stalks.

Place a large non-stick frying pan on a medium-high heat. With a sharp knife, score the sea bass skin at 2cm intervals, then rub all over with the curry paste, inside and out, getting into all the cracks and crannies. Pack the coriander stalks into the cavities, season with sea salt and black pepper, then place in the hot pan with 1 tablespoon of olive oil. Cook for 3 to 4 minutes per side, or until dark golden and cooked through (depending on the thickness of your fish).

Drain and shake off the spring onions and coriander and pile on to your plates. Sit the sea bass on top, spooning over any spicy oil from the pan. Finely grate over the lime zest, and serve with lime halves, for squeezing over.

CALORIES	FAT	SAT FAT	PROTEIN	CARBS	SUGAR	SALT	FIBRE
410kcal	28.1g	4.8g	37.4g	2.1g	1.2g	1.5g	0.2g

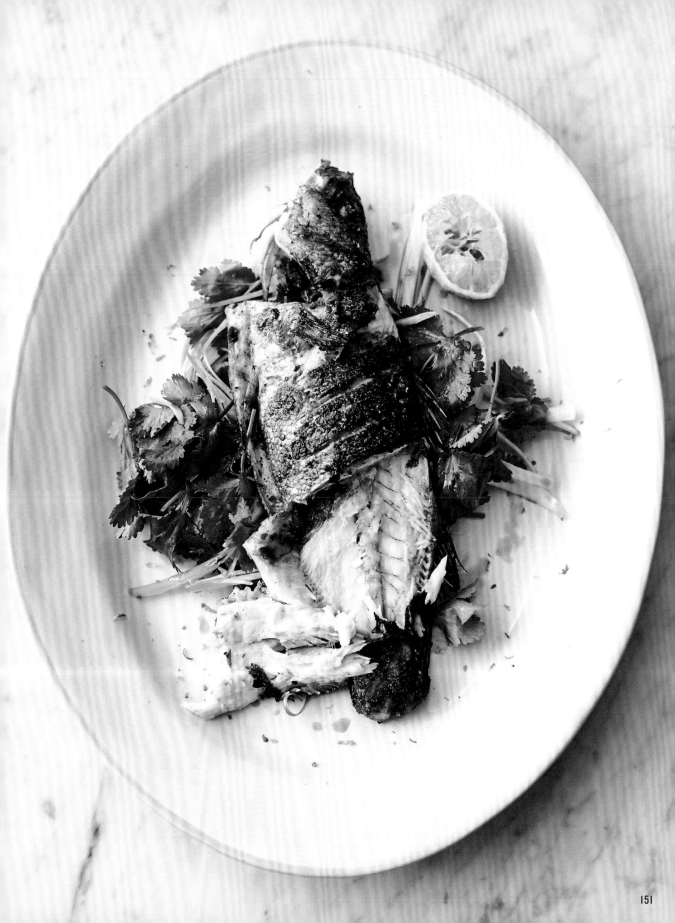

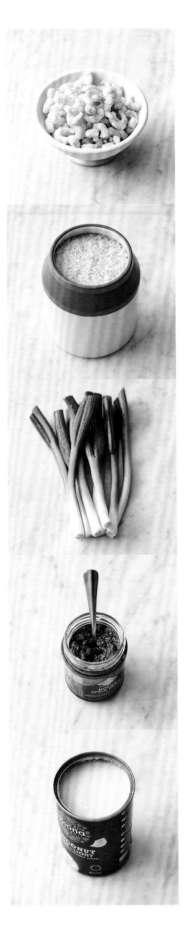

SPEEDY SPICED PRAWN SOUP

SERVES 4   TOTAL 20 MINUTES

250g small frozen cooked peeled prawns

150g basmati rice

8 spring onions

2 heaped tablespoons korma curry paste

1 x 400ml tin of light coconut milk

Place the prawns in a bowl of cold water so they start to defrost. Meanwhile, dry fry and toast the rice for 3 minutes in a large shallow casserole pan on a high heat, stirring regularly, while you trim and finely slice the spring onions. Add 1 tablespoon of olive oil, the spring onions and korma paste to the pan. Stir for 2 minutes, then pour in the coconut milk and 2½ tins' worth of water. Boil for 12 minutes, stirring everything occasionally.

With 6 minutes to go, drain the prawns, finely chop and stir into the soup. When the rice is cooked through and the soup is your desired consistency, taste, season to utter perfection with sea salt and black pepper, and dish up.

CALORIES	FAT	SAT FAT	PROTEIN	CARBS	SUGAR	SALT	FIBRE
321kcal	13.1g	6g	16.1g	36.2g	3.9g	1.2g	2g

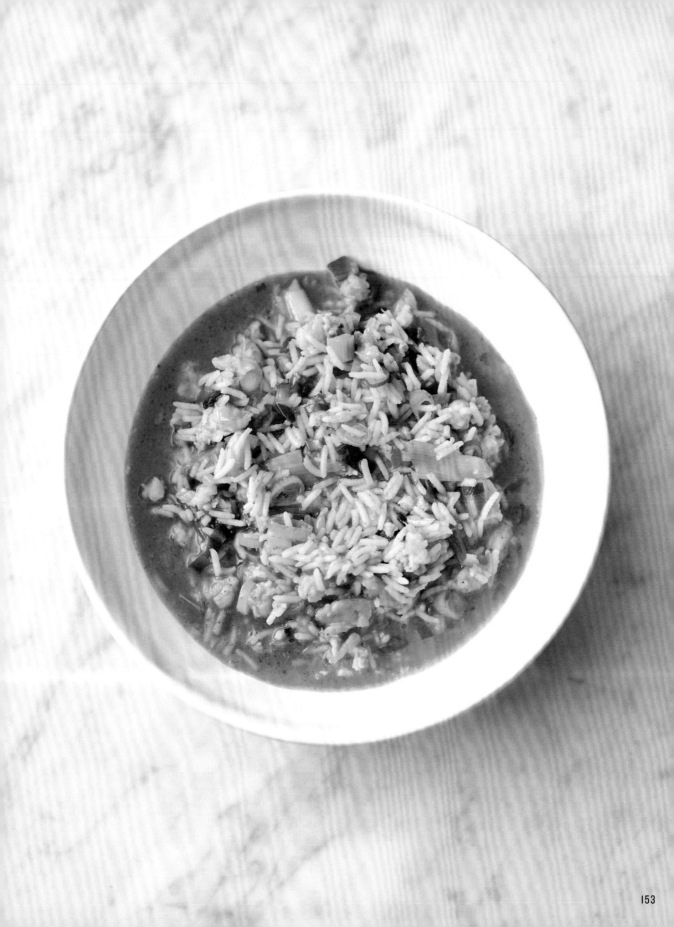

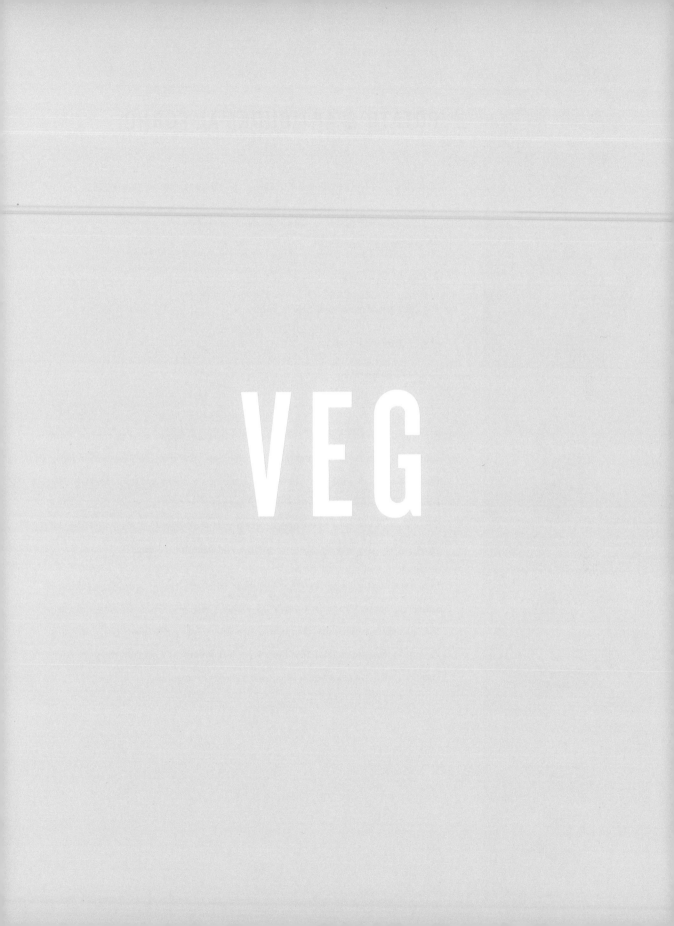
VEG

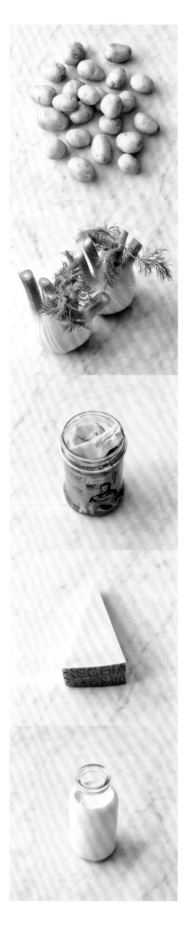

POTATO & ARTICHOKE AL FORNO

SERVES 6   FAST PREP 9 MINUTES   SLOW COOK 1 HOUR 20 MINUTES

800g baby new potatoes

2 large bulbs of fennel

1 x 280g jar of artichoke hearts in oil

50g Parmesan cheese

100ml double cream

Preheat the oven to 200°C/400°F/gas 6. Halve any larger new potatoes. Trim the fennel, pick and reserve any leafy tops, finely slice the stalky part, then halve the bulb and cut into 1cm slices. Put it all into a 30cm x 35cm roasting tray, halve the artichokes and add with 2 tablespoons of oil from their jar, as well as a really good pinch of black pepper, then toss it all together. Pour in 300ml of water, cover the tray tightly with tin foil, and bake for 1 hour.

In a bowl, finely grate half the Parmesan into the cream and loosen with a splash of water. When the time's up, remove the tray from the oven, discard the foil, spoon over the cream mixture and finely grate over the remaining Parmesan. Bake for a final 20 minutes, or until golden and cooked through, then sprinkle over any reserved fennel tops before serving.

CALORIES	FAT	SAT FAT	PROTEIN	CARBS	SUGAR	SALT	FIBRE
258kcal	14.6g	7.6g	7.3g	24.7g	4.1g	1.3g	6.3g

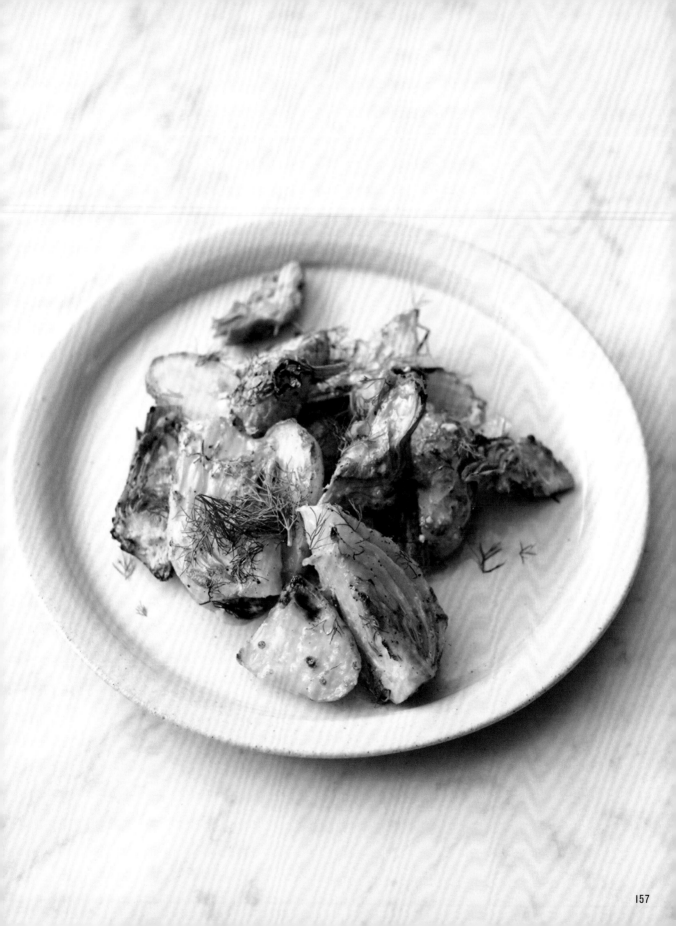

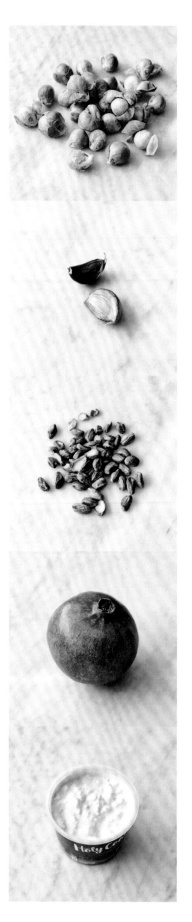

GNARLY GARLIC BRUSSELS

SERVES 2   TOTAL 16 MINUTES

300g Brussels sprouts

2 cloves of garlic

30g shelled unsalted pistachios

1 pomegranate

2 heaped tablespoons cottage cheese

Trim the sprouts, discard any tatty outer leaves, then cut in half. Place cut side down in a single layer in a large dry non-stick frying pan on a high heat, and char for 5 minutes. Meanwhile, peel and finely slice the garlic. Crush the pistachios in a pestle and mortar. Halve the pomegranate, squeeze the juice of one half through a sieve into a bowl, then hold the other half cut side down in your fingers and bash the back of it with a spoon so all the seeds tumble out. Stir the sliced garlic into the sprouts with 1 tablespoon of olive oil and a couple of splashes of water, then cook for 1 more minute.

Divide the cottage cheese between your plates, spoon the gnarly sprouts on top, then sprinkle over the pomegranate seeds and pistachios. Drizzle over the pomegranate juice and 1 tablespoon of extra virgin olive oil, sprinkle with a pinch of sea salt and black pepper from a height, and serve. Delicious.

CALORIES	FAT	SAT FAT	PROTEIN	CARBS	SUGAR	SALT	FIBRE
327kcal	25.2g	4.8g	12.8g	13g	9.4g	0.7g	1.1g

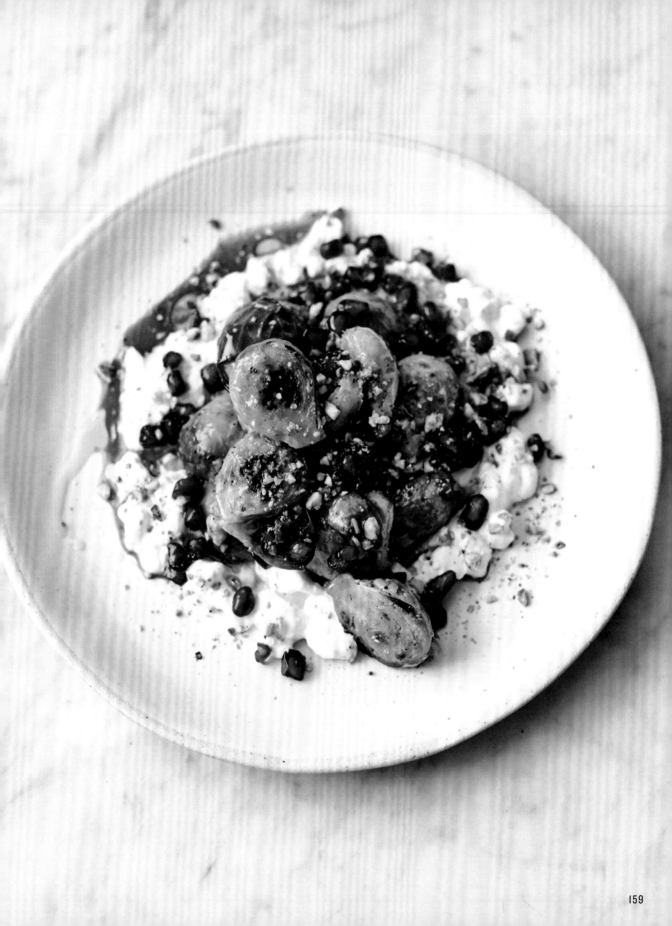

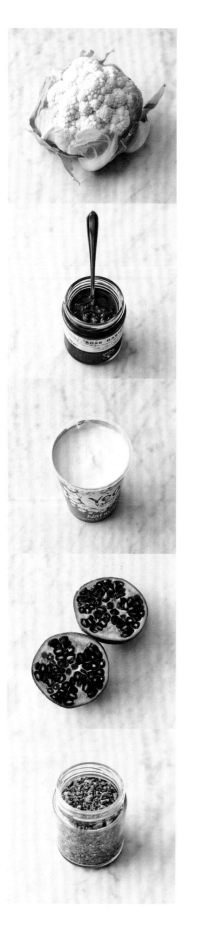

SPICED WHOLE ROAST CAULI

SERVES 2—4 | FAST PREP 9 MINUTES | SLOW COOK 1 HOUR 25 MINUTES

1 small head of cauliflower (600g)

2 heaped teaspoons rose harissa

2 heaped tablespoons natural yoghurt

1 pomegranate

1 tablespoon dukkah

Preheat the oven to 180°C/350°F/gas 4. Discard any tough outer leaves from the cauliflower, then, keeping it whole, use a sharp knife to carefully slice a cross deep into the stalk so you can easily portion it up later. In a bowl, mix together the harissa, yoghurt, ½ a tablespoon of red wine vinegar and a little sea salt and black pepper, then quickly rub the mixture all over the cauli. Place it in a snug-fitting ovenproof frying pan or roasting tray. Halve the pomegranate and squeeze the juice of one half through a sieve over the cauli. Add 100ml of water at the base, and roast for 1 hour 15 minutes.

When the time's up, baste the cauli with the juices in the pan, then return to the oven for a final 10 minutes. Remove the pan, spoon the juices back over the cauli, then quickly sprinkle over the dukkah so it sticks. Holding the remaining pomegranate half cut side down in your fingers, bash the back of it with a spoon so all the seeds tumble over the cauli, then halve or quarter, and dish up.

CALORIES	FAT	SAT FAT	PROTEIN	CARBS	SUGAR	SALT	FIBRE
181kcal	6.8g	1.9g	13.7g	16.1g	13.7g	0.6g	6.8g

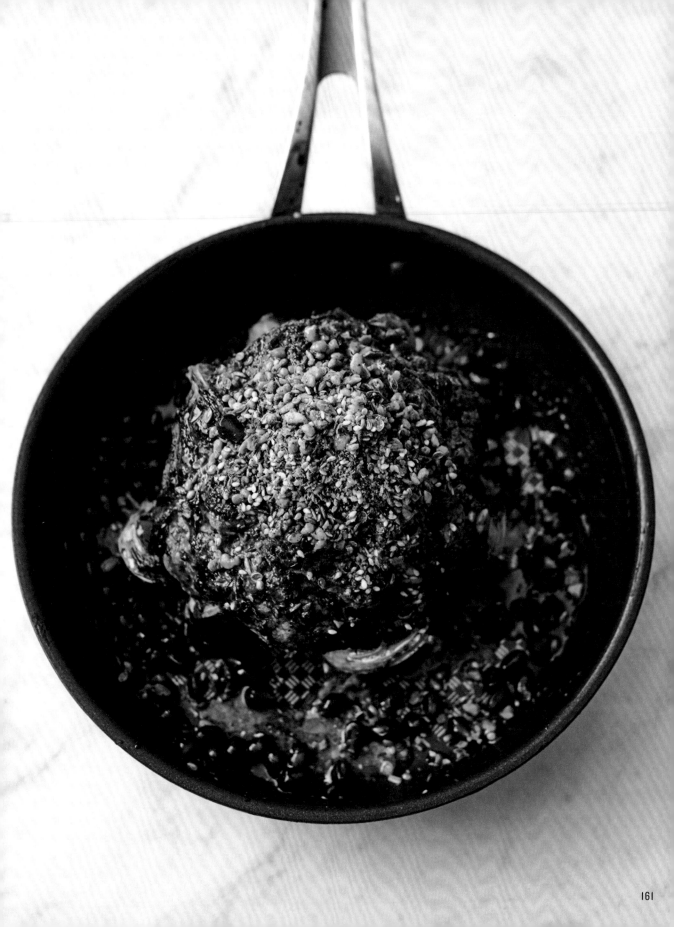

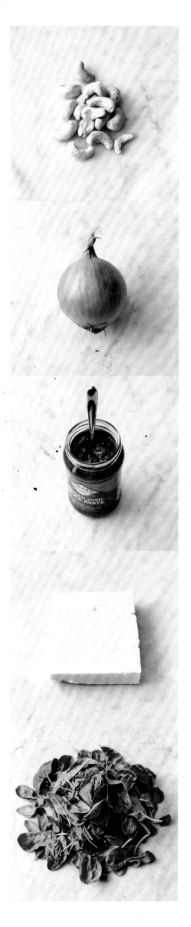

SPEEDY SPINACH CURRY

SERVES 2   TOTAL 16 MINUTES

20g unsalted cashew nuts

1 onion

2 teaspoons rogan josh curry paste

100g paneer cheese

200g baby spinach

Put a large non-stick frying pan on a medium-high heat and toast the cashew nuts as it heats up, shaking the pan occasionally until lightly golden. Tip the cashews into a pestle and mortar, returning the pan to the heat.

Peel and finely slice the onion and place in the hot pan with 1 tablespoon of olive oil and the curry paste. Cook and stir for 8 minutes, then add 1 tablespoon of red wine vinegar. Let the vinegar cook away for 30 seconds, dice and add the paneer, then the spinach. Stir until the spinach wilts and all the liquid evaporates, then taste and season to perfection with sea salt and black pepper. Crush the cashew nuts and sprinkle over the top before serving. Yum.

CALORIES	FAT	SAT FAT	PROTEIN	CARBS	SUGAR	SALT	FIBRE
363kcal	26.7g	9.9g	18.8g	11.7g	8.1g	0.7g	5.1g

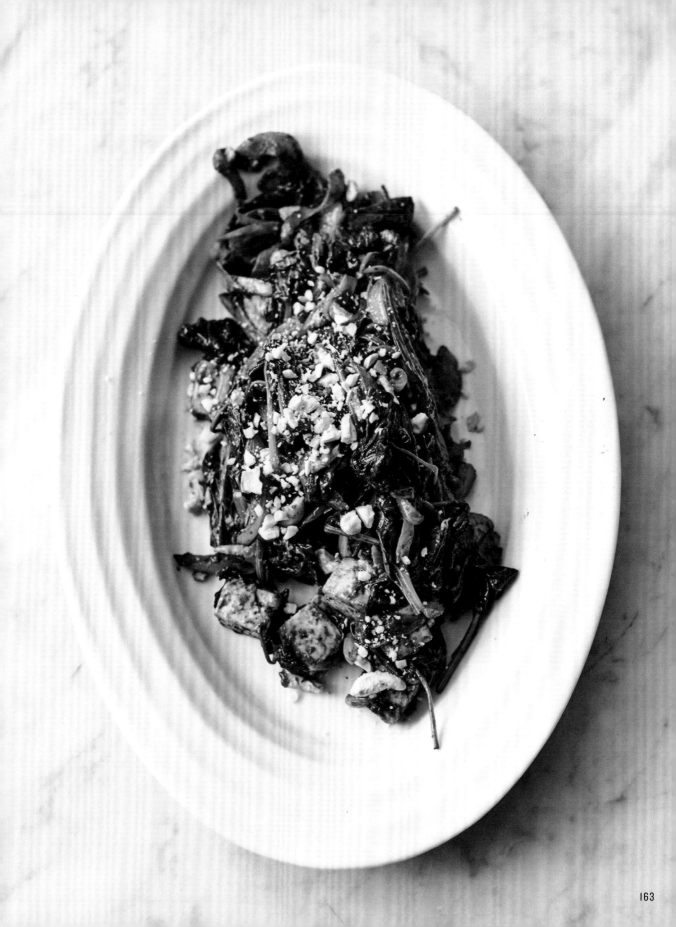

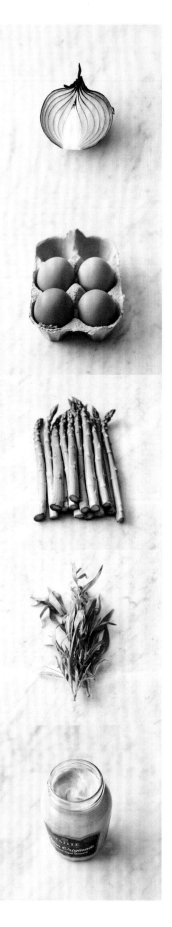

ASPARAGUS, EGGS & FRENCH DRESSING

SERVES 2 | TOTAL JUST 15 MINUTES

½ a small red onion

4 large eggs

350g asparagus

½ a bunch of fresh tarragon (15g)

2 heaped teaspoons Dijon mustard

Peel and very finely chop the red onion, place in a bowl, cover with 4 tablespoons of red wine vinegar and add a very good pinch of sea salt. Lower the eggs into a pan of vigorously simmering water and boil for 5½ minutes exactly. Line up the asparagus, trim off the woody ends, and place in a colander above the eggs, covered, to steam while the eggs cook. Meanwhile, pick the tarragon leaves.

In a bowl, whisk the mustard with 6 tablespoons of extra virgin olive oil, adding it gradually, then pour in the soaking vinegar from the onion through a sieve, whisking constantly. Taste and season to perfection with black pepper.

When the time's up on the eggs, divide the asparagus between your plates. Refresh the eggs under cold water until cool enough to handle, then peel, halve and plate up, sprinkled with the tarragon leaves and onion. Drizzle each plate with 1 tablespoon of dressing (save the rest for another day), season from a height with a pinch of pepper, and dig in.

CALORIES	FAT	SAT FAT	PROTEIN	CARBS	SUGAR	SALT	FIBRE
302kcal	22.7g	4.8g	19.7g	6g	4.9g	0.9g	3.5g

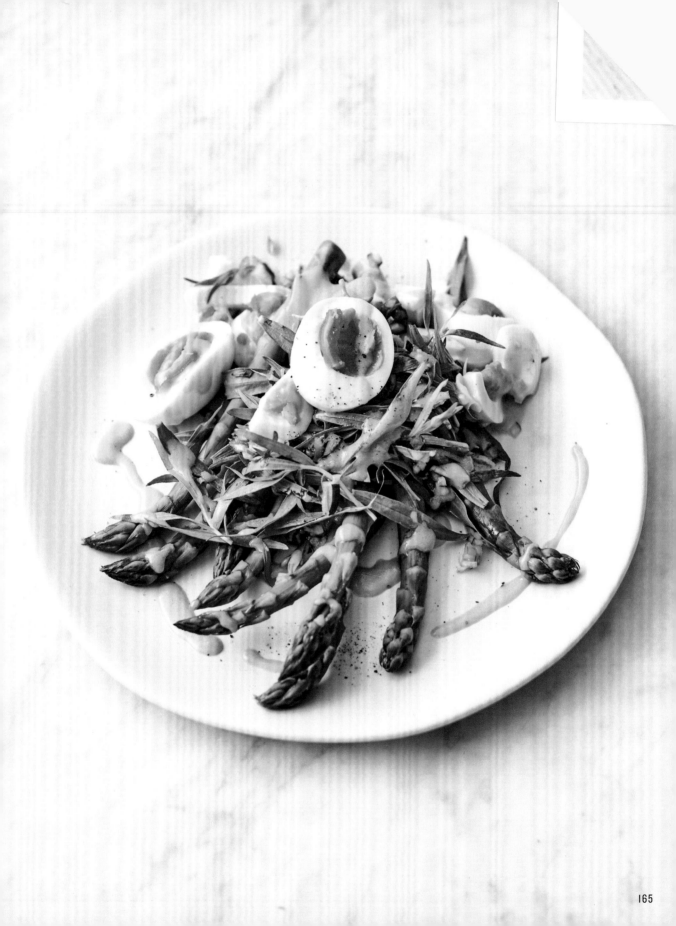

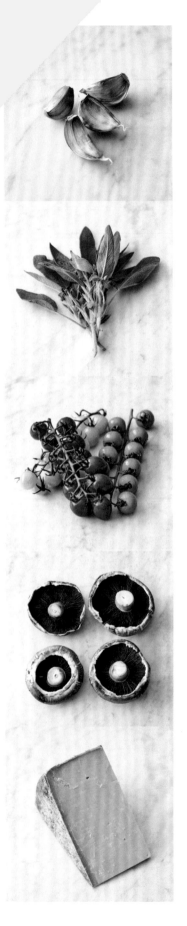

BAKED GARLICKY MUSHROOMS

SERVES 2   TOTAL 30 MINUTES

4 cloves of garlic

½ a bunch of fresh sage (15g)

350g ripe mixed-colour cherry tomatoes

4 large portobello mushrooms

40g Cheddar cheese

Preheat the oven to 200°C/400°F/gas 6. Peel and very finely slice the garlic. Pick the sage leaves. Halve the cherry tomatoes. Peel the mushrooms, reserving the peel. Place it all (peel included) in a 25cm x 30cm roasting tray and drizzle with 1 tablespoon each of olive oil and red wine vinegar. Add a pinch of sea salt and black pepper and toss together. Pick out 12 perfect garlic slices and sage leaves for later, and sit the mushrooms stalk side up on the top. Bake for 10 minutes.

Remove the tray from the oven, crumble the cheese into the mushroom cups and sprinkle over the reserved garlic and sage. Return to the oven for 15 more minutes, or until the cheese is melted and everything's golden, then dish up.

CALORIES	FAT	SAT FAT	PROTEIN	CARBS	SUGAR	SALT	FIBRE
211kcal	15.2g	5.8g	10.1g	8.9g	5.9g	0.9g	3.4g

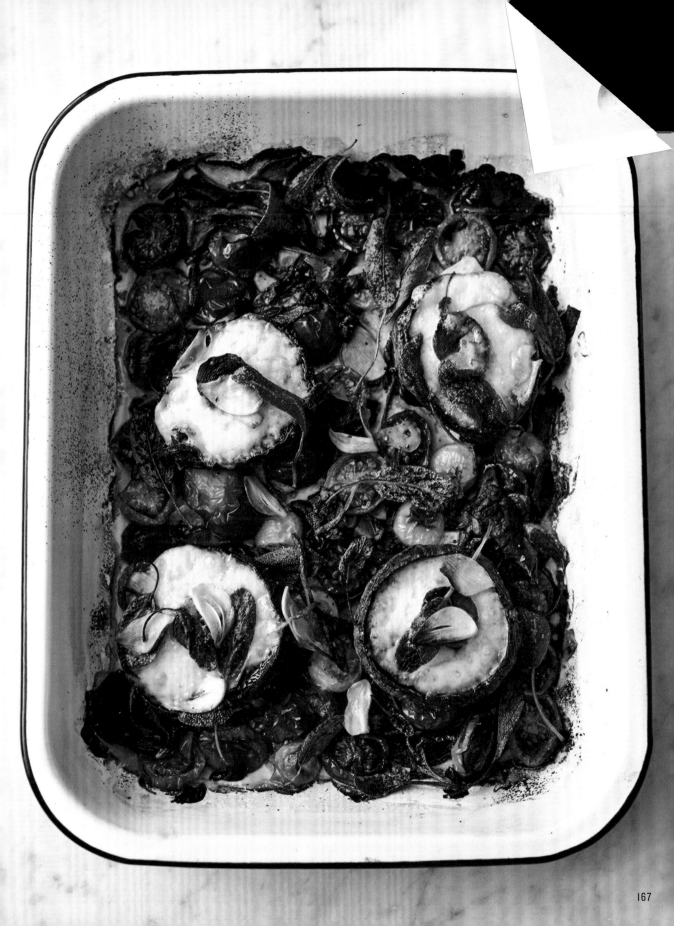

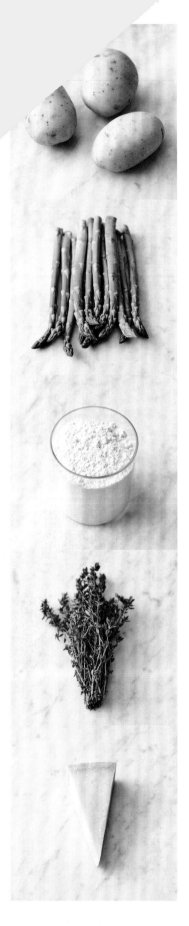

EASY RUSTIC GNOCCHI

SERVES 2 | TOTAL 30 MINUTES

400g floury potatoes

350g asparagus

50g plain flour

½ a bunch of fresh thyme (15g)

50g Parmesan cheese

Wash the potatoes, chop into 3cm chunks and cook in a large pan of boiling salted water for 12 minutes, or until tender. Meanwhile, line up the asparagus, trim off the woody ends, then slice the stalks 1cm thick, leaving the tips whole.

Drain the potatoes and steam dry for 2 minutes, then return to the pan and mash well. Taste and season to perfection with sea salt and black pepper, then tip on to a clean work surface. Fill the empty pan with boiling kettle water and place on a high heat. Use your hands to scrunch the flour with the potato, then divide into 24 pieces. Squeeze each in your palm to compress, into little uneven gnocchi, then drop into the boiling water for 1 minute, or until they float.

Meanwhile, put the asparagus into a large non-stick frying pan on a medium-low heat with 1 tablespoon of olive oil, stirring occasionally. Strip in most of the thyme leaves, then use a slotted spoon to add the gnocchi straight in. Finely grate over most of the Parmesan and toss well, adding 100ml of gnocchi cooking water to emulsify it into a nice sauce. Taste, season to perfection, then dish up. Grate over the remaining Parmesan, strip over the remaining thyme, and finish with a little drizzle of extra virgin olive oil.

CALORIES	FAT	SAT FAT	PROTEIN	CARBS	SUGAR	SALT	FIBRE
434kcal	16g	6g	21.3g	54.5g	6g	0.5g	6.4g

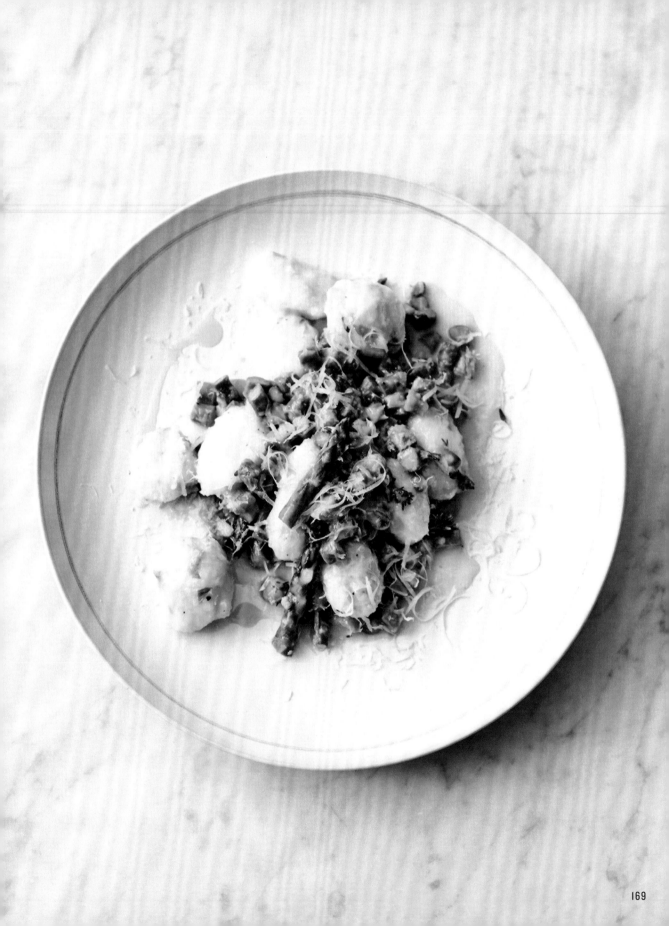

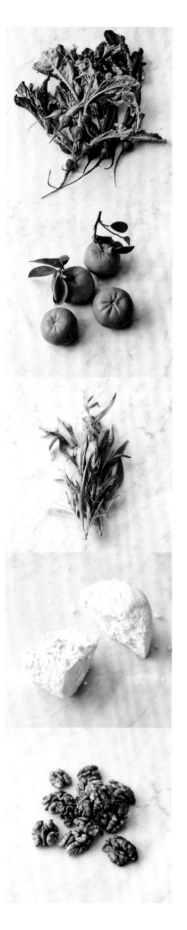

AMAZING DRESSED BEETS

SERVES 4   TOTAL 27 MINUTES

600g raw mixed-colour baby beets, ideally with leaves

4 clementines

½ a bunch of fresh tarragon (15g)

100g crumbly goat's cheese

40g shelled unsalted walnut halves

Reserving any nice smaller beet leaves, halve any larger beets and cook, covered, in a pan of boiling salted water for 15 to 20 minutes, or until tender. Meanwhile, squeeze the juice of 1 clementine into a large bowl with 1 tablespoon of extra virgin olive oil and a good splash of red wine vinegar. Peel the remaining 3 clementines, slice into fine rounds and arrange on your plates.

Drain the beets and briefly refresh in cold water until cool enough to quickly rub off the skins. Halve or slice a few, then toss them all in the dressing. Taste, season to perfection with sea salt and black pepper, then pick in the tarragon and toss with the reserved beet leaves. Divide between your plates, crumble over the goat's cheese and walnuts, and drizzle lightly with extra virgin olive oil.

CALORIES	FAT	SAT FAT	PROTEIN	CARBS	SUGAR	SALT	FIBRE
263kcal	18.1g	5.9g	9.8g	16.1g	14.9g	0.6g	3.7g

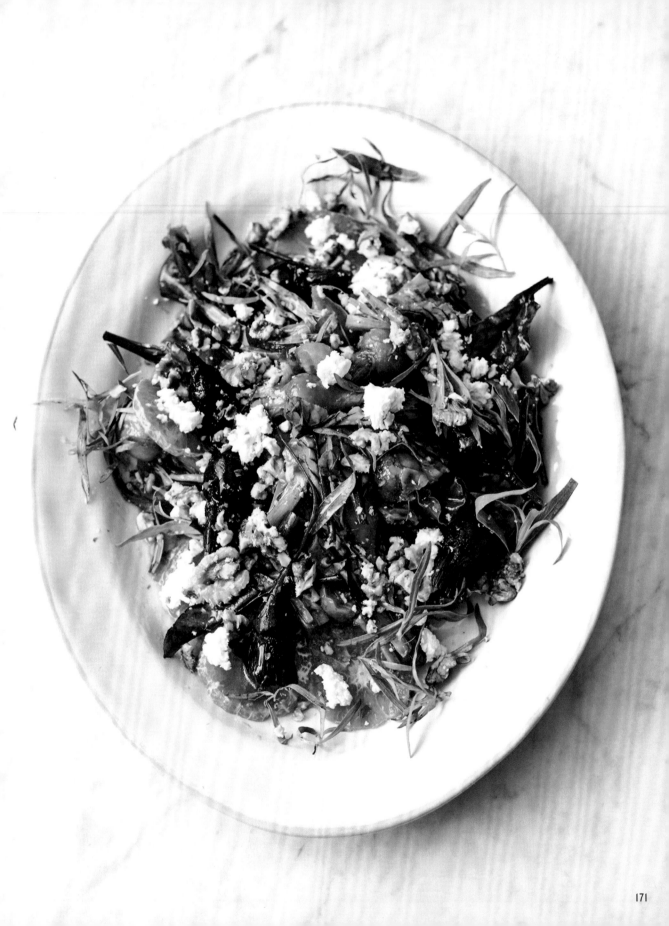

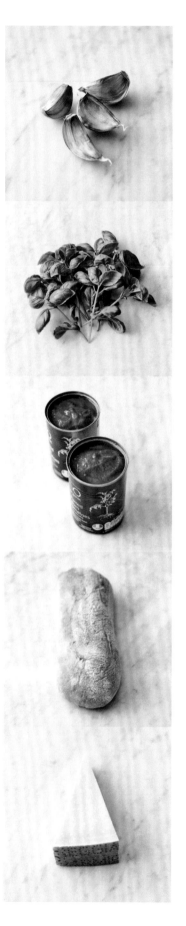

PAPPA AL POMODORO SOUP

SERVES 4   TOTAL 21 MINUTES

4 cloves of garlic

1 bunch of fresh basil (30g)

2 x 400g tins of plum tomatoes

270g stale ciabatta

40g Parmesan cheese

Peel and finely slice the garlic, and place in a large pan on a medium heat with 1 tablespoon of olive oil, stirring regularly. Pick the baby basil leaves into a bowl of cold water for later, then pick the rest of the leaves into the pan. Before the garlic starts to colour, add the tomatoes and 2 tins' worth of water, season with sea salt and black pepper, and bring to the boil, gently mashing the tomatoes.

Tear in the stale bread, stir, then leave to simmer on a low heat for 5 minutes, or until thick and delicious. Finely grate and stir in the Parmesan, then taste and season to perfection. Dish up, sprinkle over the reserved baby basil leaves and drizzle each bowlful with 1 tablespoon of good extra virgin olive oil. Heaven.

CALORIES	FAT	SAT FAT	PROTEIN	CARBS	SUGAR	SALT	FIBRE
357kcal	15.5g	3.7g	13.3g	44g	9.9g	1.3g	3.8g

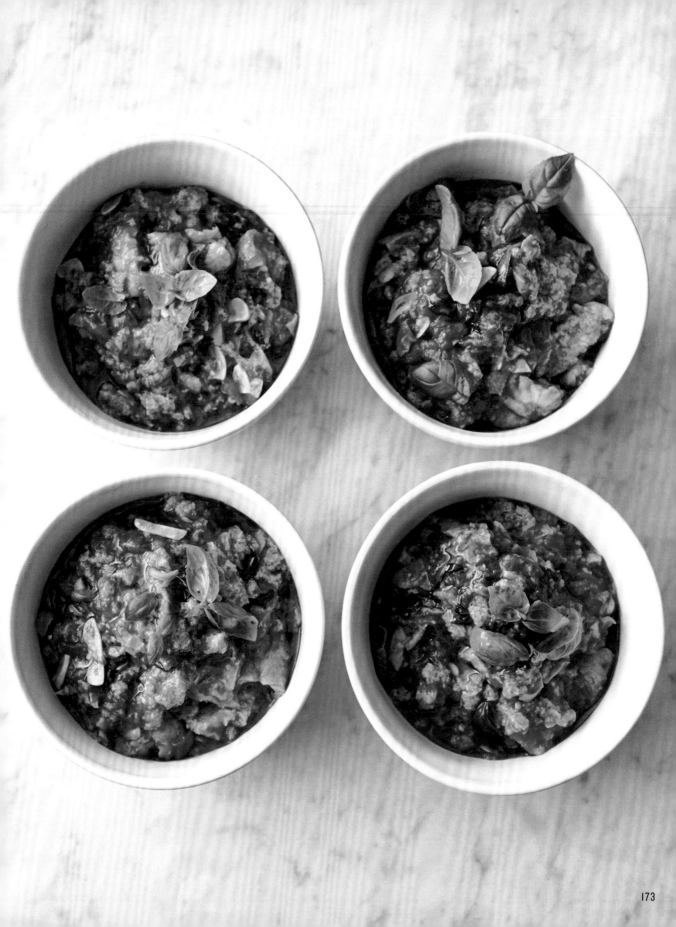

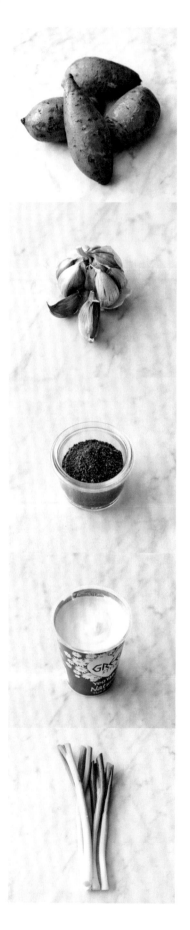

CAJUN SWEET POTATOES

SERVES 4   FAST PREP 9 MINUTES   SLOW COOK 1 HOUR

4 sweet potatoes (250g each)

1 bulb of garlic

1 heaped teaspoon Cajun spice

200ml Greek yoghurt

4 spring onions

Preheat the oven to 180°C/350°F/gas 4. Quickly scrub the sweet potatoes clean, then slice into 3cm rounds. Place in a 25cm x 30cm roasting tray with the whole unpeeled garlic bulb, and toss with 1 tablespoon each of olive oil and red wine vinegar, a pinch of sea salt and black pepper and the Cajun spice. Arrange in a flat layer and roast for 1 hour, or until soft, gnarly and caramelized.

Once done, squeeze all the soft, sweet, creamy, mild roasted garlic out of the skins into the yoghurt, mash together, then taste and season to perfection. Trim and finely slice the spring onions. Spoon the yoghurt across a plate or platter, stack the sweet potato on top, drizzle with ½ a tablespoon of extra virgin olive oil, sprinkle over the spring onions, dish up and daddy dance.

CALORIES	FAT	SAT FAT	PROTEIN	CARBS	SUGAR	SALT	FIBRE
346kcal	10.6g	4g	6.6g	59.7g	18.6g	1.1g	0.1g

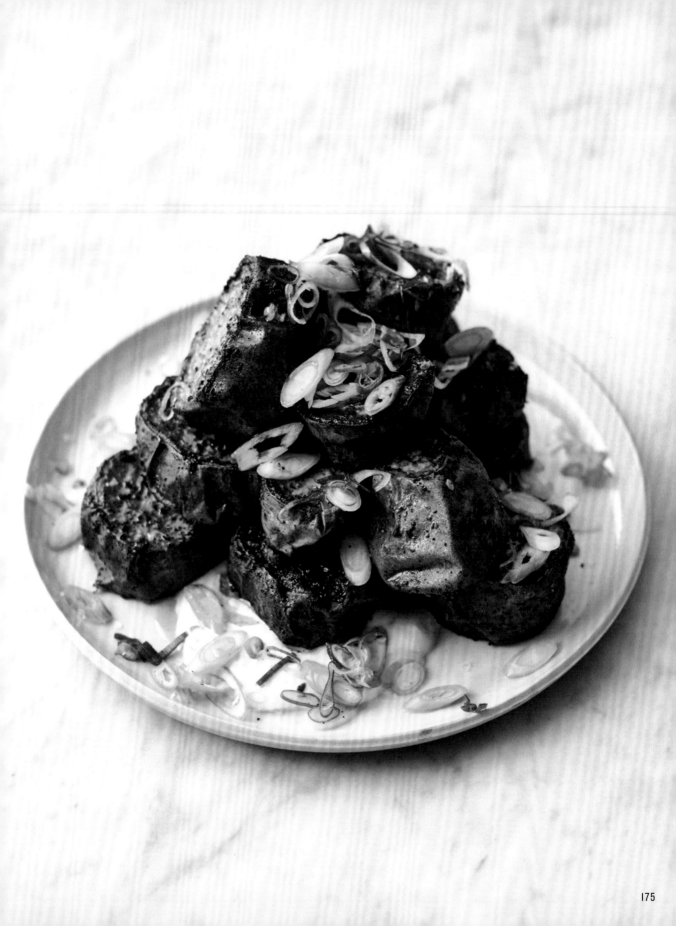

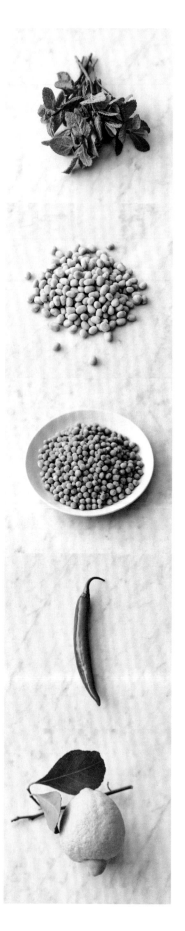

PEAS, BEANS, CHILLI & MINT

SERVES 2—4   TOTAL JUST 10 MINUTES

½ a bunch of fresh mint (15g)

200g fresh podded or frozen broad beans

200g fresh podded or frozen peas

1 fresh red chilli

1 lemon

Rip off and reserve the top leafy half of the mint. Put the stalks in a pan of boiling salted water, then add the beans and peas to cook for 4 minutes. Meanwhile, halve and deseed the chilli and finely chop with the top leafy half of the mint. Place in a bowl, finely grate over a little lemon zest, then squeeze in all the juice. Add 2 tablespoons of extra virgin olive oil, mix, taste and season to perfection with sea salt and black pepper.

Drain the beans and peas, reserving a mugful of cooking water and discarding the mint stalks. Pinch the skins off any larger beans, then pour the beans and peas on to a platter, toss with a few splashes of reserved cooking water, then spoon over the dressing. Drizzle with 1 more tablespoon of extra virgin olive oil and toss together at the table before tucking in.

CALORIES	FAT	SAT FAT	PROTEIN	CARBS	SUGAR	SALT	FIBRE
209kcal	20.4g	3.2g	13.1g	19.5g	4.2g	0.5g	11.7g

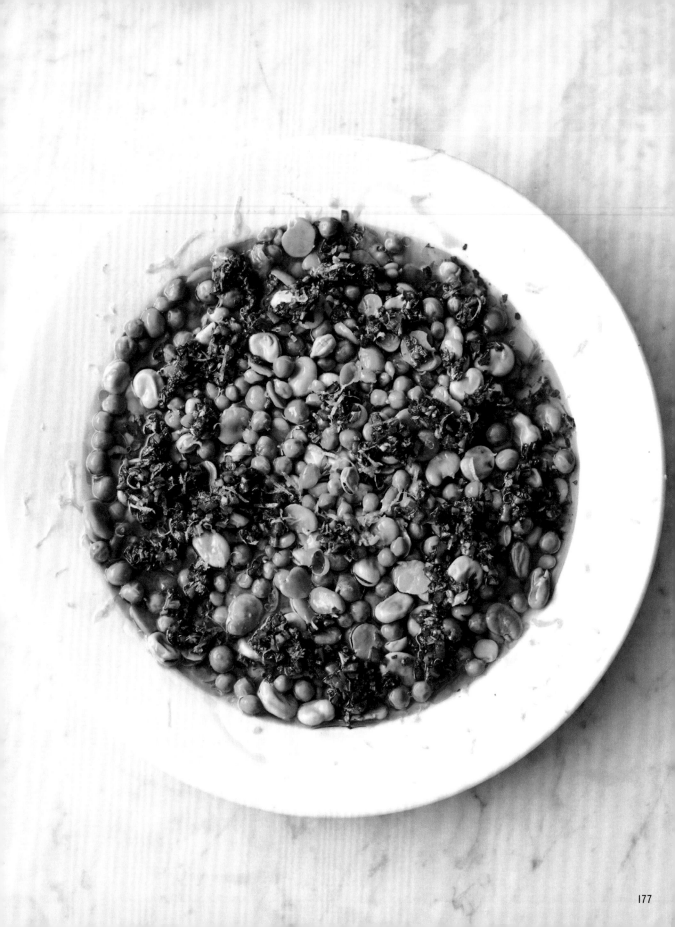

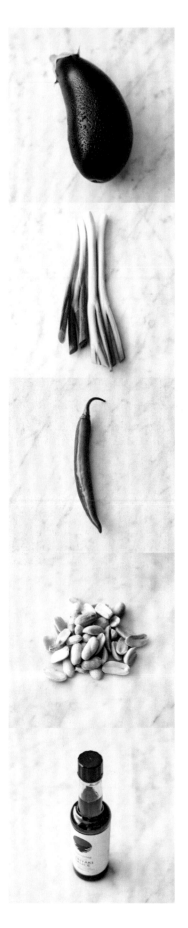

STICKY TERIYAKI AUBERGINE

SERVES 2   TOTAL 20 MINUTES

1 large aubergine (400g)

4 spring onions

1 fresh red or yellow chilli

20g unsalted peanuts

2 tablespoons teriyaki sauce

Put a 26cm non-stick frying pan on a high heat and pour in 250ml of water. Halve the aubergine lengthways, quickly slash the flesh side of each half a few times and place skin side up in the pan, then season with sea salt and black pepper. Cover and cook for 10 minutes, or until it boils dry and begins to sizzle (listen for the change in sound). Meanwhile, trim the spring onions. Cut the whites into 3cm lengths at an angle and put aside. Deseed the chilli and finely slice lengthways with the green part of the spring onions. Place both in a bowl of ice-cold water and put aside to crisp up.

When the aubergine starts to sizzle, add 1 tablespoon of olive oil, the white spring onion and the peanuts to the pan, stirring regularly. After 2 minutes, add a splash of water, drizzle in the teriyaki and reduce to a medium heat. Turn the aubergine, jiggle the pan and let it get sticky for a few minutes, then dish up, sprinkled with the drained green spring onion and chilli.

CALORIES	FAT	SAT FAT	PROTEIN	CARBS	SUGAR	SALT	FIBRE
181kcal	12g	2g	5.2g	13.3g	11.1g	1.4g	0g

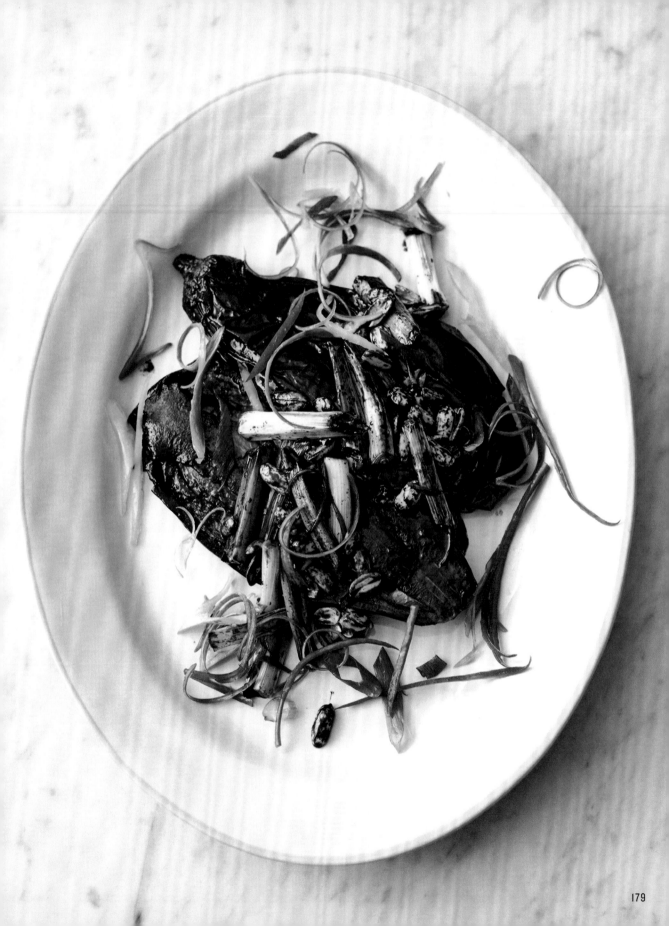

BEEF

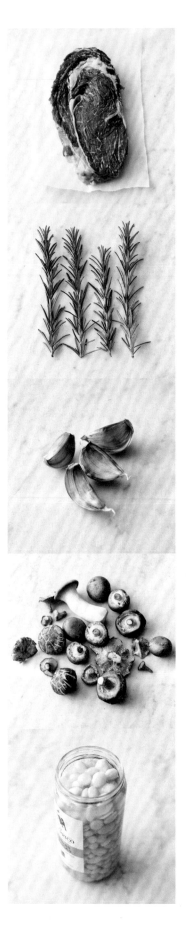

EPIC RIB-EYE STEAK

SERVES 4   TOTAL 26 MINUTES

600g piece of rib-eye steak (ideally 5cm thick), fat removed

4 sprigs of fresh rosemary

4 cloves of garlic

350g mixed mushrooms

1 x 660g jar of white beans

Place a large non-stick frying pan on a medium-high heat. Rub the steak all over with a pinch of sea salt and black pepper, then sear on all sides for 10 minutes in total, so you achieve good colour on the outside but keep it medium rare in the middle, or cook to your liking, turning regularly with tongs.

Meanwhile, strip the rosemary leaves off the sprigs, peel and finely slice the garlic, and tear up any larger mushrooms. When the steak's done, remove to a plate and cover with tin foil. Reduce the heat under the pan to medium, and crisp up the rosemary for 30 seconds, then add the garlic and mushrooms and cook for 8 minutes, or until golden, tossing regularly. Pour in the beans and their juice, add 1 tablespoon of red wine vinegar and simmer for 5 minutes, then season to perfection. Sit the steak on top and pour over any resting juices. Slice and serve at the table, finishing with a little extra virgin olive oil, if you like.

CALORIES	FAT	SAT FAT	PROTEIN	CARBS	SUGAR	SALT	FIBRE
501kcal	30.8g	13.6g	37.3g	19.7g	1.8g	0.7g	6.3g

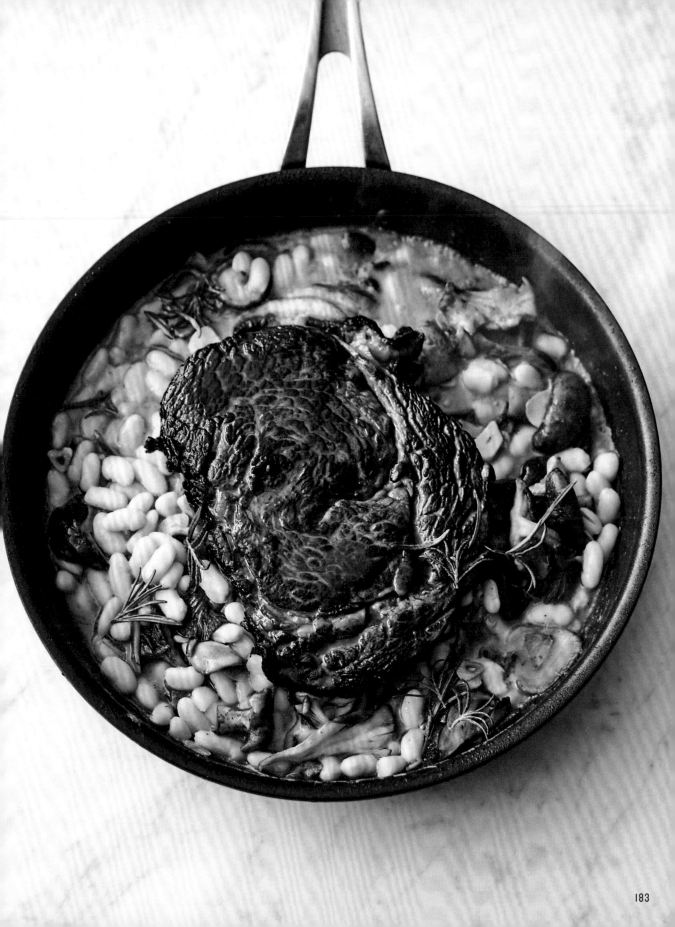

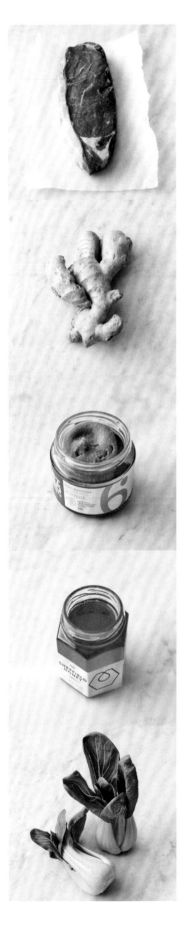

GINGER SHAKIN' BEEF

SERVES 2   TOTAL 16 MINUTES

300g sirloin steak (ideally 1.5cm thick)

4cm piece of ginger

1 tablespoon miso paste

2 teaspoons runny honey

2 pak choi (250g)

Pull the fat off the sirloin, finely slice the fat and place it in a cold non-stick frying pan. Put on a medium-high heat to crisp up while you peel and matchstick the ginger, then add that to crisp up, too. Cut off the sinew, then dice the steak into 3cm chunks and toss with the miso until well coated. Scoop the crispy fat and ginger out and put aside, then add the steak chunks to the pan. Cook for 4 minutes, tossing regularly, then drizzle in the honey and 1 tablespoon of red wine vinegar. Toss for 1 more minute until shiny and sticky.

Meanwhile, halve the pak choi, cook in a pan of boiling water for just 1 minute so they retain a bit of crunch, then drain well and plate up. Spoon over the steak and sticky juices from the pan, and finish with the reserved crispy bits.

CALORIES	FAT	SAT FAT	PROTEIN	CARBS	SUGAR	SALT	FIBRE
373kcal	19.8g	8.4g	35.7g	13.4g	9.9g	1.1g	2.9g

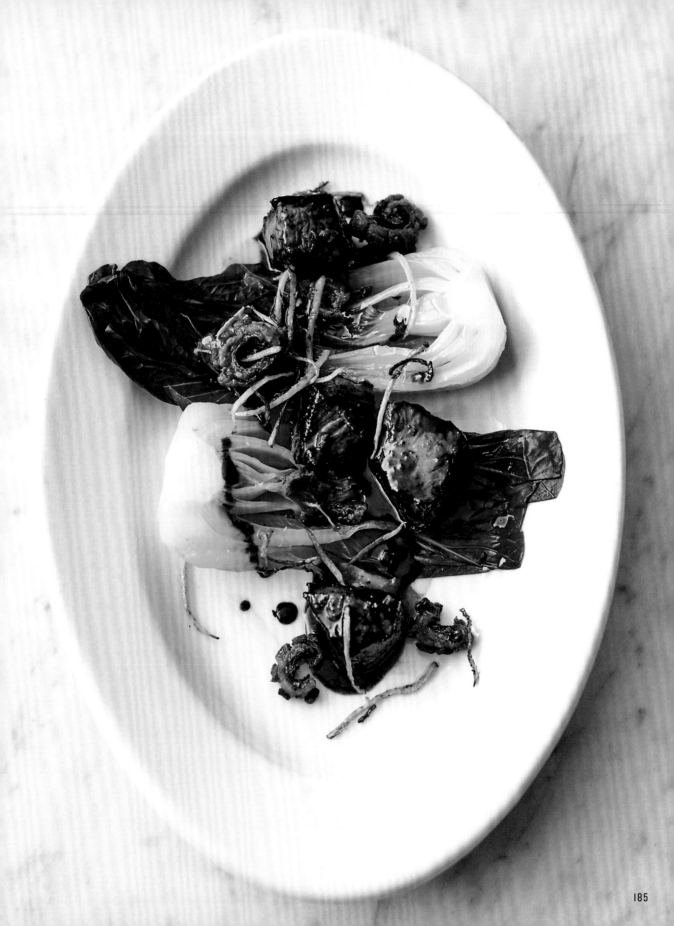

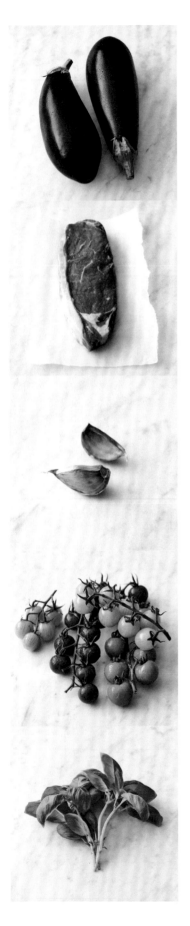

SIZZLING SIRLOIN

SERVES 2   TOTAL 30 MINUTES

2 large aubergines (800g total)

300g sirloin steak (ideally 1.5cm thick)

2 cloves of garlic

300g ripe mixed-colour cherry tomatoes

½ a bunch of fresh basil (15g)

Prick the aubergines, then microwave in a covered bowl on high for 10 minutes, or until soft. Meanwhile, pull the fat off the sirloin and place the fat in a large cold non-stick frying pan. Put on a medium-high heat to render as it heats up, moving it around to coat the pan, while you cut off the sinew, then rub the steak with a pinch of sea salt and black pepper. Peel and finely slice the garlic, and halve the tomatoes.

Sear the steak in the hot pan for 2 minutes on each side for medium, or to your liking, then remove to a plate to rest, discarding the piece of fat. Sprinkle the garlic straight into the pan. Discard the aubergine stalks, chop up the flesh and add to the pan with any tasty juices, then toss in the tomatoes for 2 minutes. Tear in most of the basil leaves, stir in 1 tablespoon of red wine vinegar, taste and season to perfection, and plate up.

Slice the steak, place on top, pick over the remaining basil, then drizzle with 1 teaspoon of extra virgin olive oil and the resting juices.

CALORIES	FAT	SAT FAT	PROTEIN	CARBS	SUGAR	SALT	FIBRE
386kcal	22.1g	9g	36.5g	11g	9.5g	0.8g	1.9g

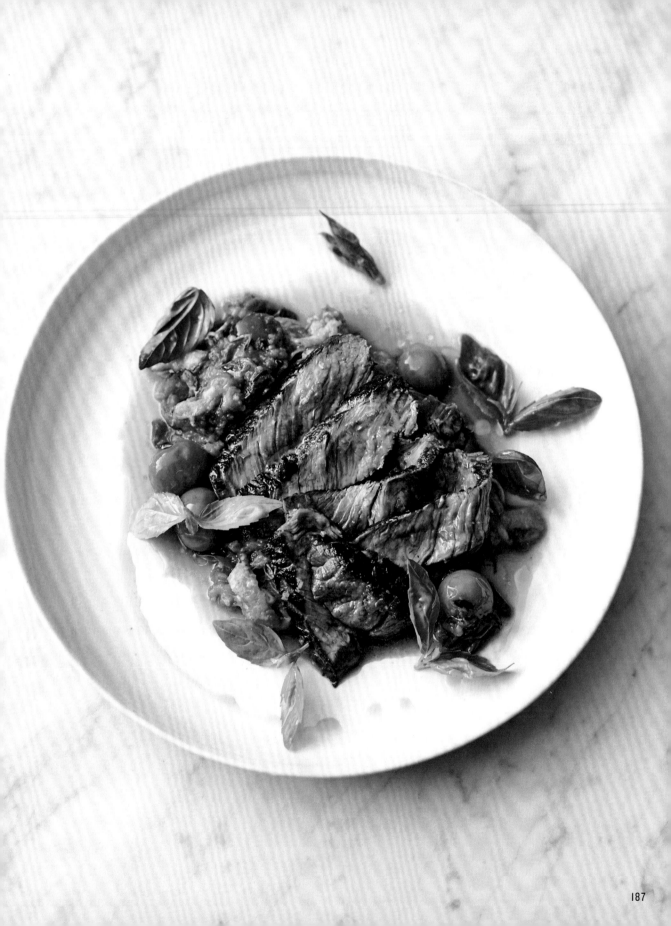

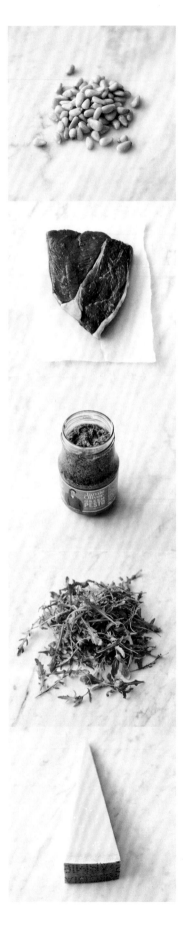

ITALIAN SEARED BEEF

SERVES 2   TOTAL JUST 10 MINUTES

1 tablespoon pine nuts

250g rump steak

2 heaped teaspoons green pesto

40g rocket

15g Parmesan cheese

Put a large non-stick frying pan on a high heat, toasting the pine nuts as it heats up, tossing regularly and removing when golden. Cut the fat off the rump, finely chop the fat and place in the pan to render and crisp up while you cut the sinew off the rump, then season it with sea salt and black pepper. Place between two sheets of greaseproof paper and bash to 1cm thick with a rolling pin, also tenderizing the meat. Scoop out and reserve the crispy bits of fat, then sear the steak in the hot pan for 1 minute on each side, until golden but still blushing in the middle. Remove to a board.

Spread the pesto over a sharing platter. Thinly slice the steak at an angle, then plate up. Pile the rocket on top, then scatter over the pine nuts and reserved crispy fat, if you like. Mix the steak resting juices with 1 tablespoon of extra virgin olive oil and drizzle over. Shave over the Parmesan, tossing before serving.

CALORIES	FAT	SAT FAT	PROTEIN	CARBS	SUGAR	SALT	FIBRE
321kcal	21.1g	5.3g	32.2g	0.7g	0.5g	1g	0.3g

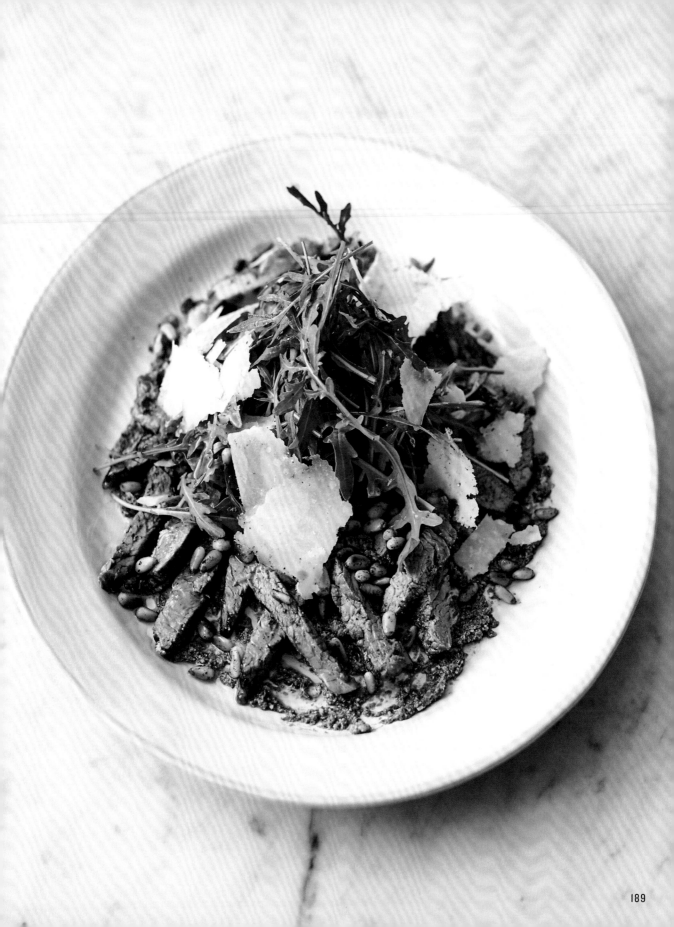

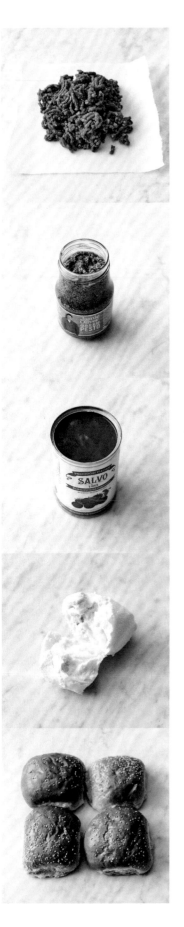

MESSY MEATBALL BUNS

SERVES 4   TOTAL 21 MINUTES

400g lean minced beef

8 heaped teaspoons green pesto

1 x 400g tin of plum tomatoes

1 x 125g ball of mozzarella

4 soft burger buns

Use your clean hands to scrunch the minced beef with half the pesto and a pinch of sea salt and black pepper. Split into 12 pieces and, with wet hands, roll into balls. Brown the balls all over in a non-stick frying pan on a high heat with 1 tablespoon of olive oil, shaking the pan regularly.

Once the balls are golden and gnarly, pour in the tomatoes, breaking them up with a wooden spoon, along with just a quarter of a tin's worth of water. Bring to the boil, slice the mozzarella and lay over the balls, pop the lid on and leave to thicken for 5 minutes on a medium heat. Meanwhile, warm your buns in a large dry non-stick frying pan or in the oven on a low heat.

Split each bun and spread 1 heaped teaspoon of pesto inside. Divvy up the balls and mozzarella with a little sauce, serving the rest on the side for dunking.

CALORIES	FAT	SAT FAT	PROTEIN	CARBS	SUGAR	SALT	FIBRE
495kcal	24g	8.5g	35.5g	35.5g	5.8g	2g	2.4g

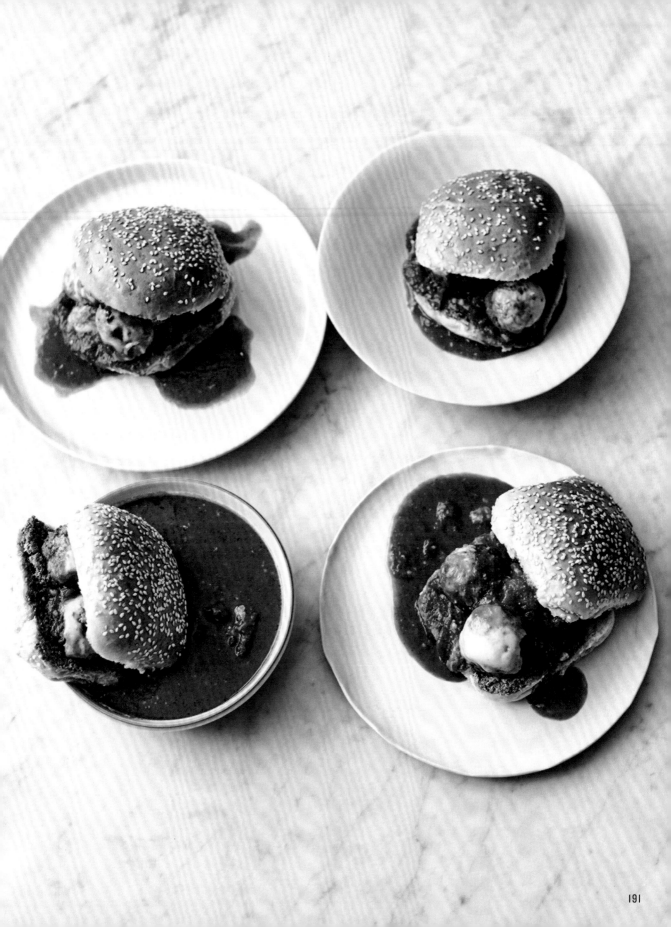

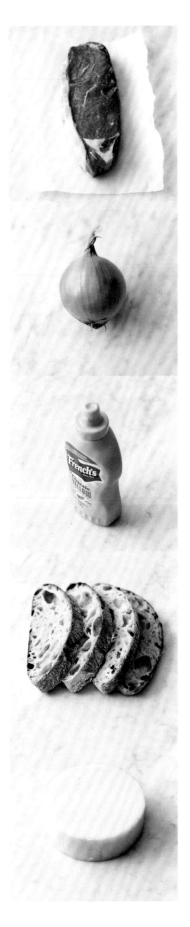

STEAK SANDWICH

SERVES 2   TOTAL JUST 14 MINUTES

250g sirloin steak (ideally 1.5cm thick)

1 large onion

2 teaspoons American mustard

4 slices of nice bread (50g each)

50g provolone or fontina cheese

Pull the fat off the sirloin, finely slice the fat and place it in a large cold non-stick frying pan. Put on a medium-high heat to render as it heats up, moving it around to coat the pan, while you peel and slice the onion into 1cm-thick rounds. Add them to the pan to char for 10 minutes, turning halfway. Meanwhile, cut off the sinew, then place the steak between two sheets of greaseproof paper and pound with your fist until just under 1cm thick. Sprinkle with a pinch of sea salt and black pepper, then brush all over with the mustard and cut into two.

Add a good splash of red wine vinegar to the onion, toss for 1 minute over the heat, then divide between two slices of bread, leaving the pan on the heat. Sear the steaks in the screaming hot pan for just 40 seconds on each side, then slice and lay over the cheese, cover, turn the heat off and leave to melt for just 40 seconds more. Lay the steak on top of the onion, pop the other slices of bread on top, drizzle with a little extra virgin olive oil, and devour.

CALORIES	FAT	SAT FAT	PROTEIN	CARBS	SUGAR	SALT	FIBRE
635kcal	25.5g	12.6g	42.3g	59.4g	8.5g	2.9g	3.4g

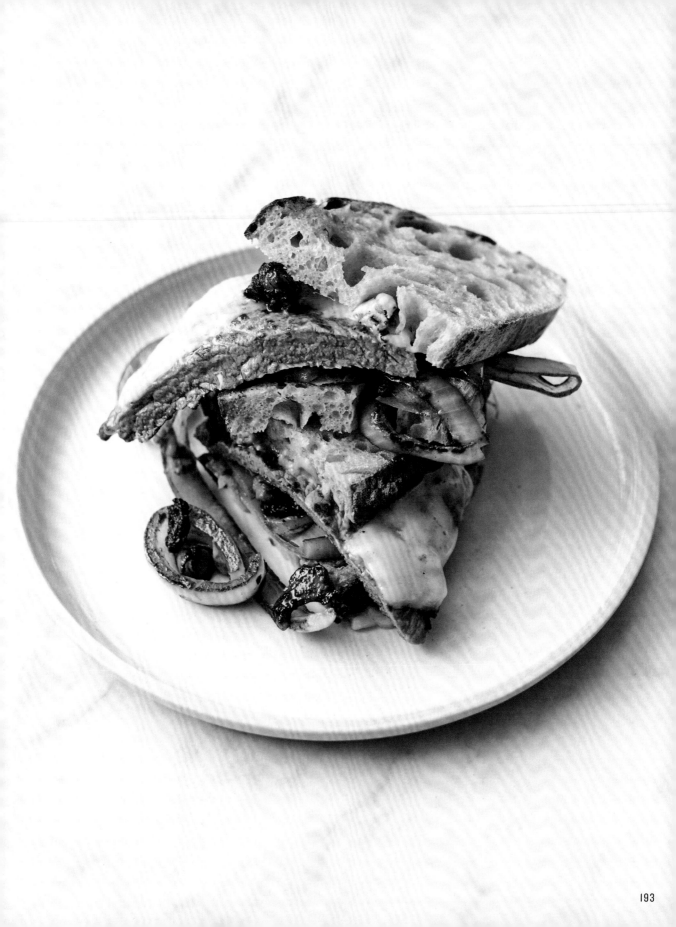

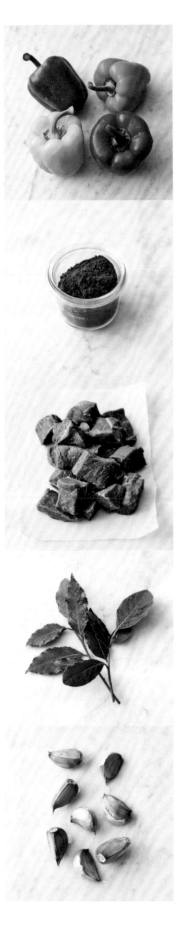

BANGIN' BEEF STEW

SERVES 4   FAST PREP 9 MINUTES   SLOW COOK 2 HOURS

4 mixed-colour peppers

1 heaped teaspoon allspice

600g lean stewing beef

10 fresh bay leaves

8 cloves of garlic

Preheat the oven to 160°C/325°F/gas 3. Place a large shallow casserole pan on a high heat. Deseed the peppers and chop into fingers, then place in the pan with 1 tablespoon of olive oil, a pinch of sea salt and black pepper and the allspice. Chop the beef a similar size and stir into the pan with the bay. Crush in the unpeeled garlic through a garlic crusher and fry for 2 minutes, tossing regularly.

Add 2 tablespoons of red wine vinegar and 500ml of water to the pan. Cover, then cook in the oven for 2 hours, or until dark and sticky. Loosen with a splash of water, if needed, mix up, taste, season to perfection, and serve.

CALORIES	FAT	SAT FAT	PROTEIN	CARBS	SUGAR	SALT	FIBRE
264kcal	9.2g	2.8g	36.2g	9.8g	6.8g	0.8g	3.6g

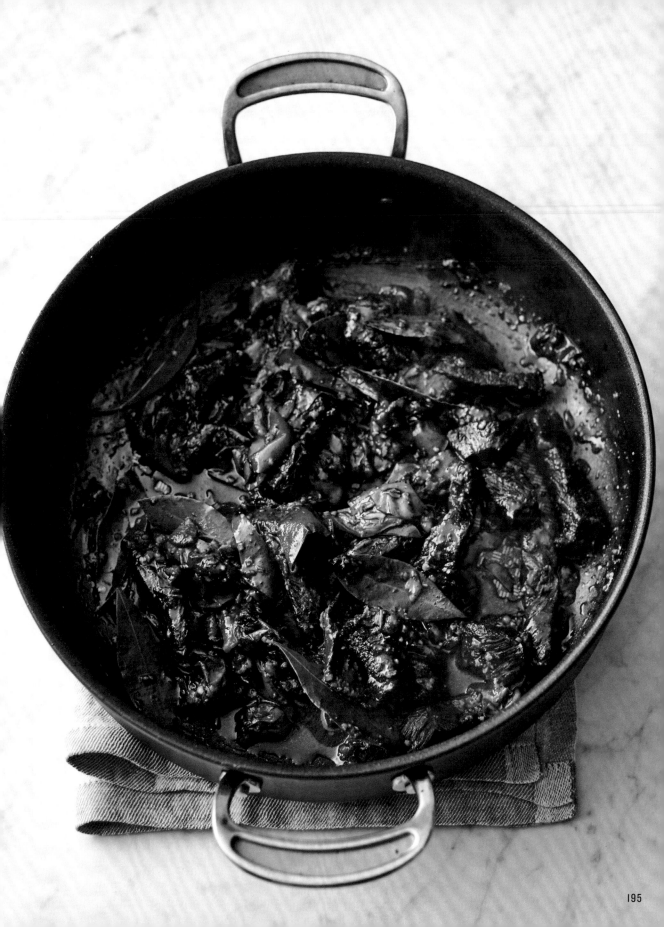

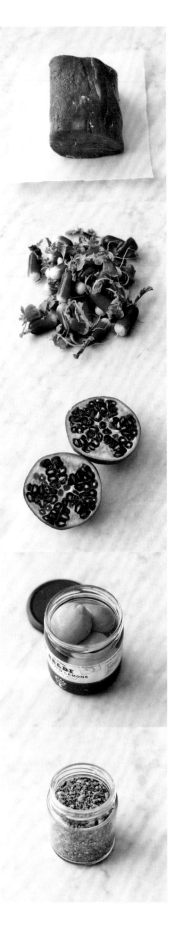

DUKKAH BEEF CARPACCIO

SERVES 4 OR 8　　TOTAL JUST 12 MINUTES

500g piece of fillet steak

300g radishes, ideally with leaves

1 pomegranate

2 preserved lemons (20g each)

1 heaped tablespoon dukkah

Rub the steak all over with ½ a tablespoon of olive oil and a pinch of sea salt and black pepper. Get a non-stick frying pan hot on a high heat, then sear the steak on all sides for 3 minutes in total. Remove to a board.

Finely slice the radishes, reserving any nice leaves. Halve the pomegranate and holding one half cut side down in your fingers, bash the back of it with a spoon so all the seeds tumble out into a bowl. Squeeze the juice from the remaining half through a sieve into a separate bowl. Quarter the preserved lemons and trim away the seedy core. Finely chop the rind and add to the pomegranate juice with 1 tablespoon each of extra virgin olive oil and red wine vinegar, then taste and season to perfection.

Slice the steak as finely as you can, then use the side of your knife to flatten and stretch out each slice. Divide between your plates, sprinkle over the radishes and leaves, then spoon over the dressing. Scatter over the dukkah and pomegranate seeds, then finish with a drizzle of extra virgin olive oil.

CALORIES	FAT	SAT FAT	PROTEIN	CARBS	SUGAR	SALT	FIBRE
265kcal	15.2g	5.6g	27.3g	4.3g	3.6g	1.1g	0.8g

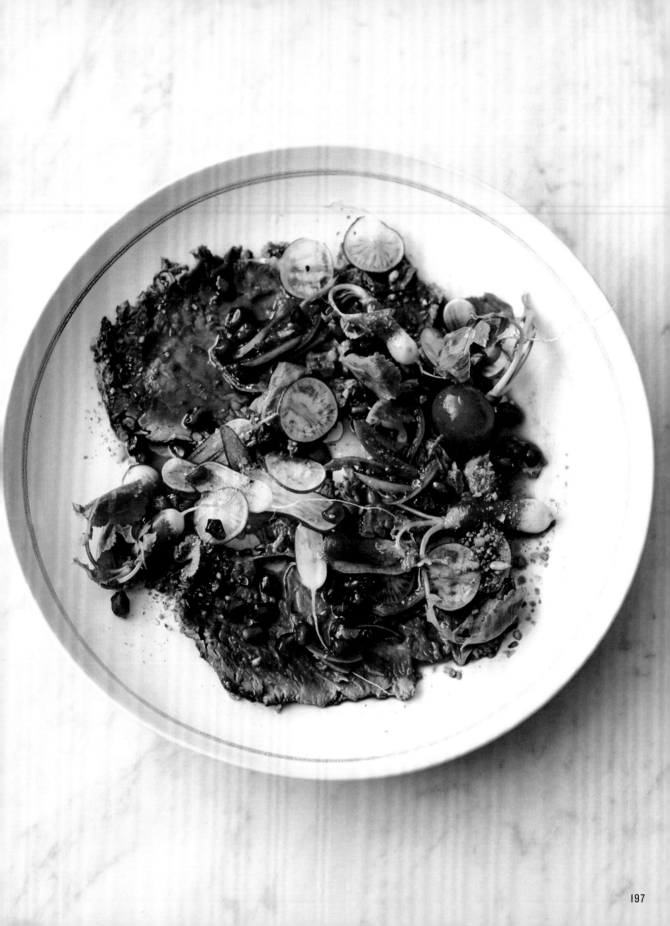

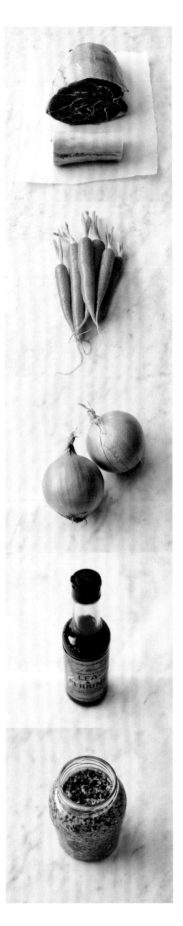

MELTIN' MUSTARDY BEEF

SERVES 6   FAST PREP 8 MINUTES   SLOW COOK 4 HOURS

900g shin of beef, bone out (ask your butcher for the bone)

500g carrots

2 onions

120ml Worcestershire sauce

2 heaped teaspoons wholegrain mustard

Preheat the oven to 160°C/325°F/gas 3. Place a large shallow casserole pan on a high heat, with a large non-stick frying pan on a high heat alongside. Dice the beef into 5cm chunks and toss with a generous amount of black pepper and a pinch of sea salt, then dry fry in the hot frying pan with the bone for 8 minutes.

Meanwhile, wash and trim the carrots, chop into 5cm chunks, and place in the casserole pan with 1 tablespoon of olive oil. Peel and quarter the onions and break apart into petals, straight into the pan, stirring regularly. When the meat is nicely coloured, tip it into the casserole pan, then stir in the Worcestershire sauce and mustard, and cover with 800ml of boiling kettle water.

Cover, then cook in the oven for 4 hours, or until the beef is meltingly tender. Loosen with a splash of water, if needed. Taste, season to perfection, and serve.

CALORIES	FAT	SAT FAT	PROTEIN	CARBS	SUGAR	SALT	FIBRE
348kcal	18g	6.4g	34g	13.4g	11.8g	1.5g	1.6g

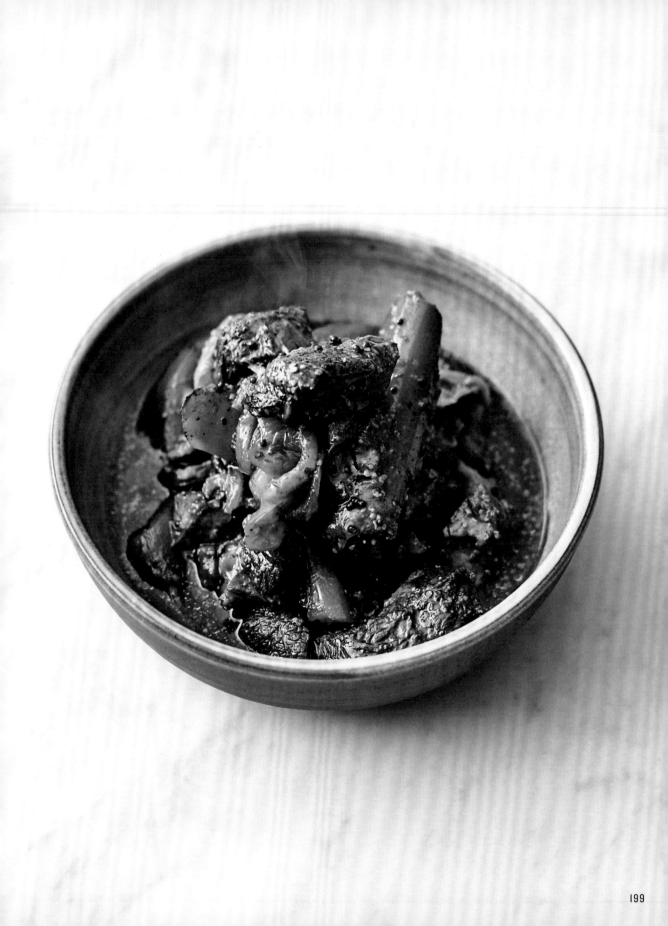

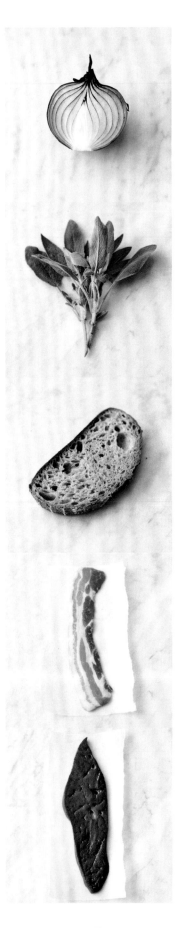

LIVER, BACON & ONIONS

SERVES 1   TOTAL JUST 15 MINUTES

½ a red onion

2 sprigs of fresh sage

1 slice of sourdough bread (50g)

1 rasher of smoked streaky bacon

125g slice of calves' liver

Peel and very finely slice the red onion. Place in a large non-stick frying pan on a medium-high heat with 1 teaspoon of olive oil. Reserving 2 nice leaves, pick, finely slice and add the rest of the sage. Cook for 5 minutes, tossing regularly.

Push the onions to one side, and add the bread and bacon to the pan. As soon as they crisp up, flip them over. Drizzle the soft, golden onions with a little red wine vinegar, toss with tongs, then move them on top of the bread, so they don't catch. Once the bacon is golden, move that on top of the onions.

Lightly season the liver, then add to the pan to sear for just 1 minute on each side, so it's golden on the outside, blushing in the middle. Add the 2 reserved sage leaves alongside, with 1 teaspoon of olive oil to crisp them up, then serve.

CALORIES	FAT	SAT FAT	PROTEIN	CARBS	SUGAR	SALT	FIBRE
362kcal	13.1g	3g	29g	32.2g	5.9g	1.1g	2.5g

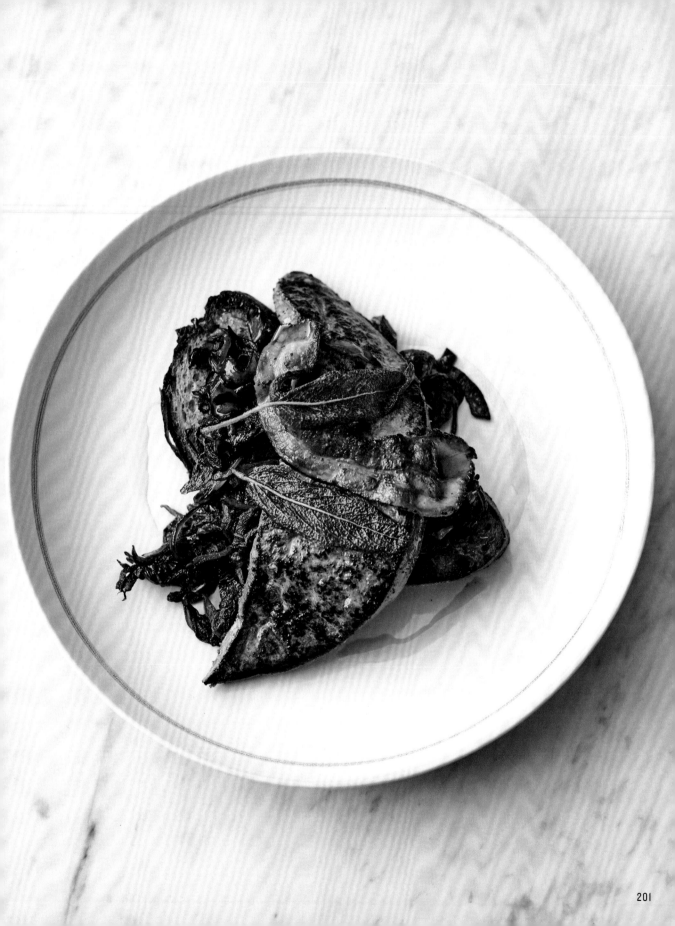

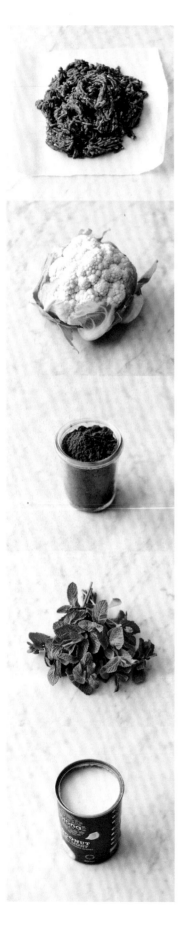

SPICY BEEF & CAULI RICE

SERVES 4   TOTAL 24 MINUTES

500g lean minced beef

1 head of cauliflower (800g)

1 heaped teaspoon rendang powder

1 bunch of fresh mint (30g)

1 x 400ml tin of light coconut milk

Place the minced beef in a large shallow casserole pan with 1 tablespoon of olive oil, then break it up and fry on a high heat, stirring regularly. Click off and discard any tatty outer leaves from the cauliflower, putting the nice leaves into a food processor. Halve the cauliflower, breaking up one half into the processor. Cut little bite-sized florets off the other half into the mince pan, chucking all the stalks into the processor as you go. Stir the rendang powder into the pan and cook it all for 10 minutes, or until crispy, stirring regularly.

Meanwhile, pick half the mint leaves into the processor, add a pinch of sea salt and black pepper, and blitz until fine. Tip into a heatproof bowl, cover, and microwave on high for 4 to 5 minutes. Reserving the baby leaves, pick the remaining mint leaves into the pan, toss well, then pour in the coconut milk and half a tin's worth of water. Bring to the boil, simmer for 5 minutes, then taste, season to perfection, and scatter over the reserved mint leaves. Give the cauli rice a good mix up, and serve on the side.

CALORIES	FAT	SAT FAT	PROTEIN	CARBS	SUGAR	SALT	FIBRE
333kcal	16g	8.5g	33.7g	12.5g	8.2g	0.9g	4.1g

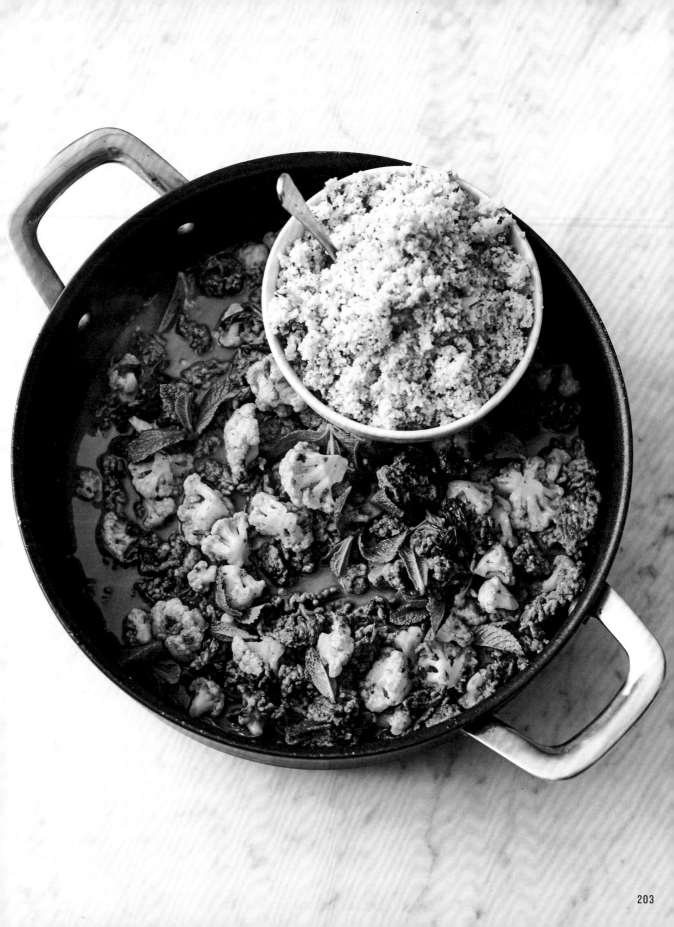

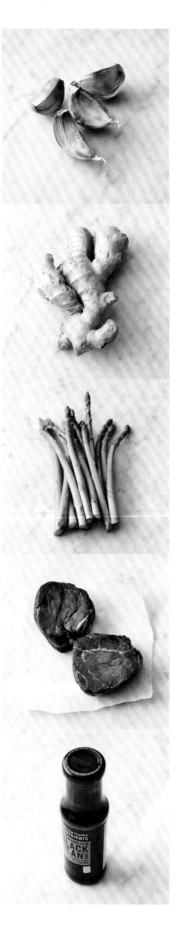

QUICK STEAK STIR-FRY

SERVES 2   TOTAL 16 MINUTES

4 cloves of garlic

4cm piece of ginger

350g asparagus

2 x 125g fillet steaks

2 tablespoons black bean sauce

Peel and very finely slice the garlic and ginger. Put into a large cold non-stick frying pan with 1 tablespoon of olive oil, and place on a medium heat, stirring regularly. Once crisp and lightly golden, scoop out of the pan and put aside, leaving the garlicky oil behind. Line up the asparagus spears and trim off the woody ends, then add the spears to the hot pan. Season the steaks with sea salt and black pepper, add alongside the asparagus and turn the heat up to high. Cook for just 3 minutes, turning everything regularly.

Toss in the black bean sauce and 1 tablespoon of red wine vinegar for 1 minute – this will give you medium-rare steaks. Alternatively, cook to your liking. Slice the steaks, dish up, then scatter over the crispy garlic and ginger.

CALORIES	FAT	SAT FAT	PROTEIN	CARBS	SUGAR	SALT	FIBRE
325kcal	17.9g	6g	32.6g	8.5g	5.1g	0.9g	0.5g

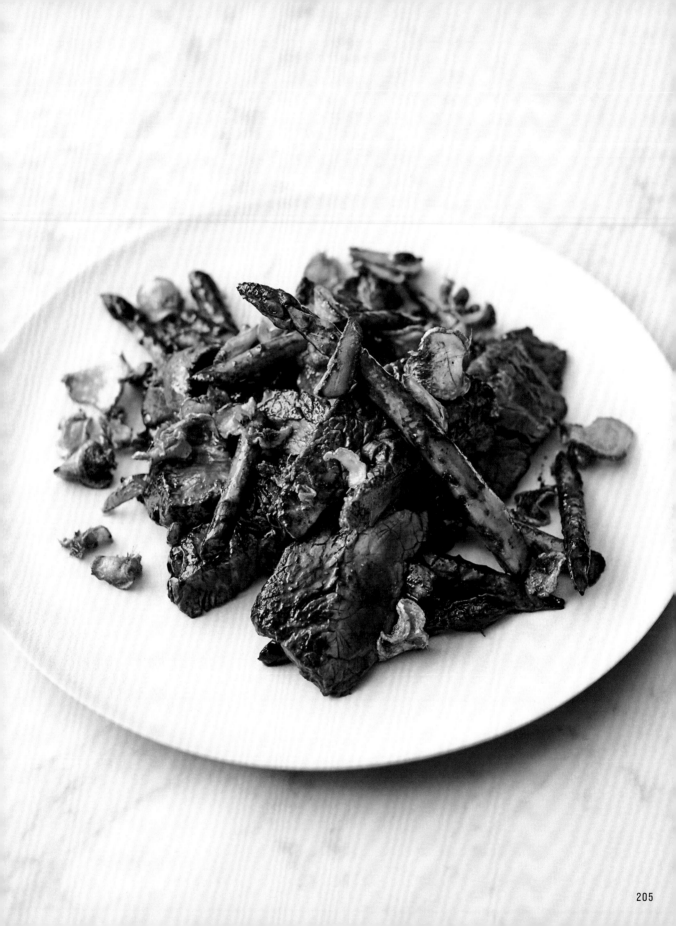

PORK

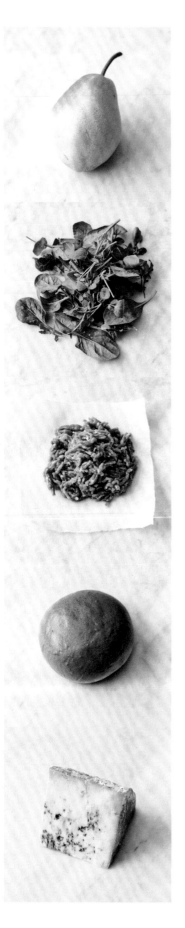

CRAZY GOOD PORK BURGER

SERVES 1 | TOTAL 16 MINUTES

1 ripe sweet pear

50g mixed spinach, rocket & watercress

150g minced pork

1 soft burger bun

30g blue cheese

Slice the pear lengthways as finely as you can. Toss gently with the salad leaves, a little drizzle each of extra virgin olive oil and red wine vinegar, and a pinch of black pepper. Scrunch the minced pork in your clean hands with a pinch of seasoning, then shape into a 1cm-thick patty. Rub with 1 teaspoon of olive oil, then place in a large non-stick frying pan on a high heat for 2 minutes, while you halve and toast the bun alongside, removing it when golden.

Flip the burger, then, after 2 minutes, crumble the blue cheese next to it to melt. Move the burger on top of the oozy cheese, jiggle around to coat, then put it on your bun base. Stack in as much pear and salad as the bun will hold, pop the lid on, squash and devour, with any extra salad on the side.

CALORIES	FAT	SAT FAT	PROTEIN	CARBS	SUGAR	SALT	FIBRE
669kcal	34.5g	12.9g	42.3g	50.7g	19.3g	2.5g	6.8g

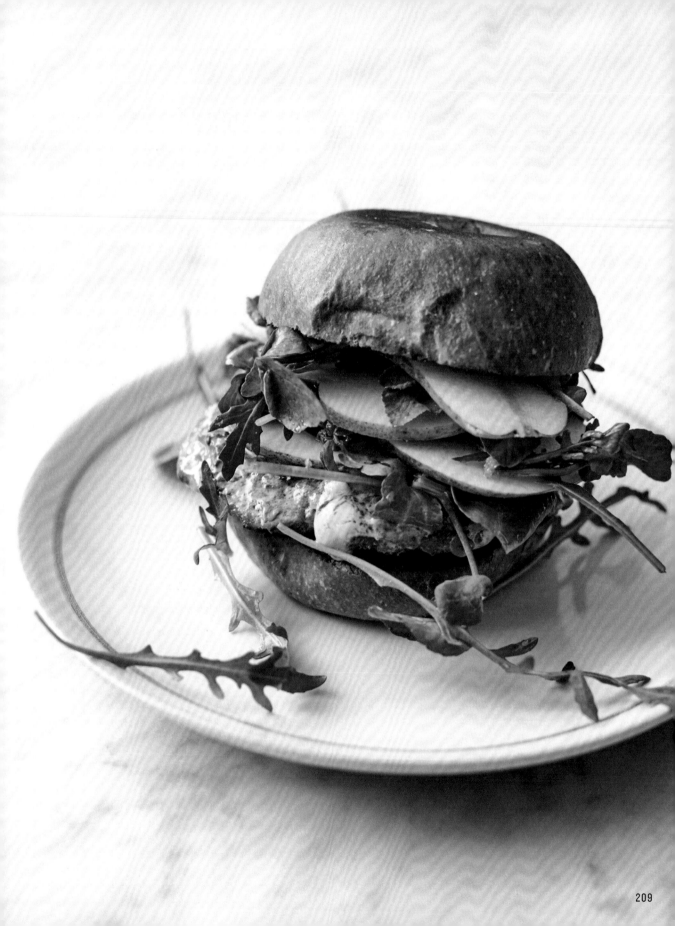

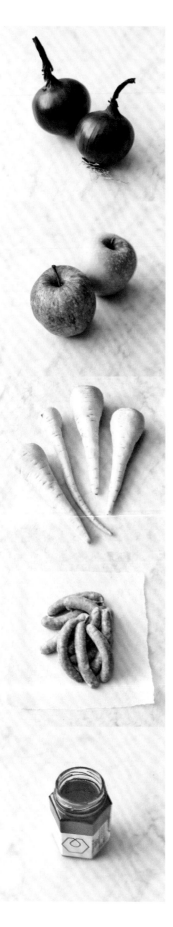

SAUSAGE & APPLE BAKE

SERVES 4   FAST PREP 9 MINUTES   COOK 35 MINUTES

2 large red onions

2 eating apples

4 parsnips

12 chipolatas

1 tablespoon runny honey

Preheat the oven to 180°C/350°F/gas 4. Place a large non-stick ovenproof frying pan on a medium-high heat. Peel the onions, cut into quarters and quickly break apart into petals directly into the pan, tossing regularly, then add 1 tablespoon of olive oil and a pinch of sea salt and black pepper. Quarter and core the apples, then toss into the pan. Use a speed-peeler to peel the parsnips into long strips. Stir 1 tablespoon of red wine vinegar into the frying pan, then pile the parsnip strips on top of the apples and onions.

Lay the sausages on top, then drizzle with 1 tablespoon of olive oil and add a pinch of black pepper from a height. Bake for 30 minutes, then drizzle over the honey and return to the oven for 5 minutes, or until golden and delicious.

CALORIES	FAT	SAT FAT	PROTEIN	CARBS	SUGAR	SALT	FIBRE
489kcal	28.8g	7.9g	22.4g	36.4g	24.8g	1.8g	10.6g

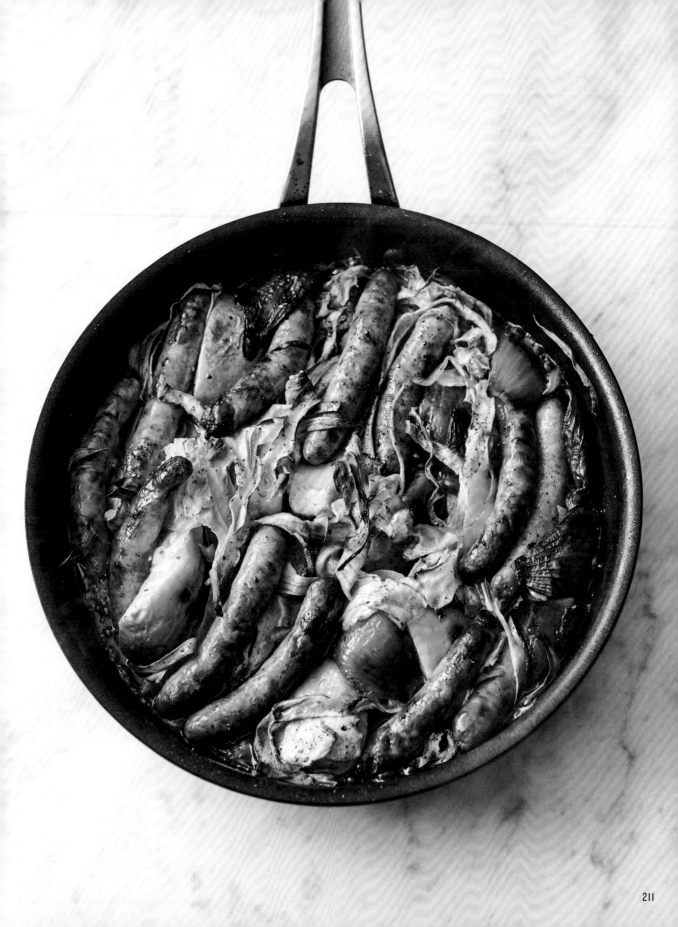

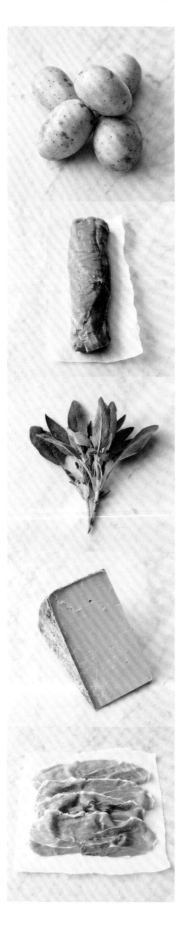

PORK & MASH GRATIN

SERVES 4 | TOTAL 30 MINUTES

800g potatoes

400g piece of pork fillet

2 sprigs of fresh sage

40g Cheddar cheese

4 slices of prosciutto

Preheat the grill to high. Wash the potatoes, chop into 3cm chunks, then cook in a large pan of boiling salted water with the lid on for 12 minutes, or until tender. Meanwhile, put a shallow casserole pan on a high heat. Season the pork with sea salt and black pepper, then place in the pan with 1 tablespoon of olive oil and sear for 3 minutes, turning regularly, while you pick the sage leaves. Remove the pork to a plate, toss the sage leaves into the fat in the pan for just 5 seconds, then scoop on to a plate, leaving the pan off the heat to use again.

Drain the spuds, tip into the casserole pan, grate over half the cheese, add 1 tablespoon of extra virgin olive oil and mash well, loosening with a splash of water, if needed. Taste, season to perfection, and spread out to the edges. Grate over the remaining cheese, sit the pork on top, then gratinate under the grill for 10 minutes. Lay the prosciutto around the pork in waves, sprinkle over the crispy sage, then grill for 2 more minutes, or until the pork is cooked to your liking. Rest for 2 minutes, then slice the pork and dish up.

CALORIES	FAT	SAT FAT	PROTEIN	CARBS	SUGAR	SALT	FIBRE
420kcal	18.4g	5.9g	31g	34.7g	1.2g	1.3g	2.6g

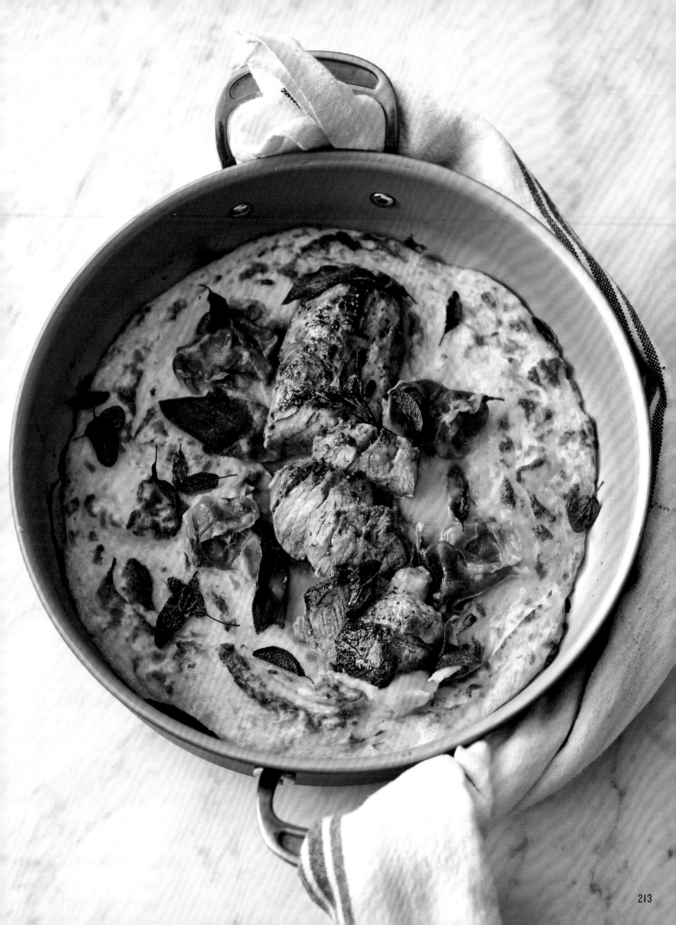

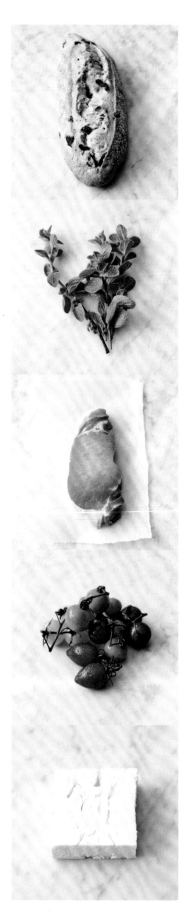

GOLDEN PORK ESCALOPE

SERVES 1   TOTAL 16 MINUTES

1 slice of olive bread (50g)

4 sprigs of fresh oregano

1 x 125g pork escalope

100g ripe mixed-colour cherry tomatoes

10g feta cheese

Blitz the bread into fine crumbs in a food processor with half the oregano leaves. Place the pork between two sheets of greaseproof paper, then bash and flatten with a rolling pin to ½cm thick. Pat the crumbs on to both sides, then bash again until they stick. Place a large non-stick frying pan on a medium-high heat and, once hot, drizzle in 1 tablespoon of olive oil. Cook the breaded escalope for 3 minutes on each side, or until dark golden.

Meanwhile, halve the tomatoes and pick the remaining oregano leaves. Transfer the escalope to your plate, wipe the pan out with a ball of kitchen paper, then add the tomatoes and remaining oregano with ½ a tablespoon of olive oil and 1 tablespoon of red wine vinegar. Toss for 1 minute, taste, season to perfection with sea salt and black pepper, then dish up and crumble over the feta.

CALORIES	FAT	SAT FAT	PROTEIN	CARBS	SUGAR	SALT	FIBRE
540kcal	28.5g	5.6g	43.8g	26g	4.9g	1.4g	4.2g

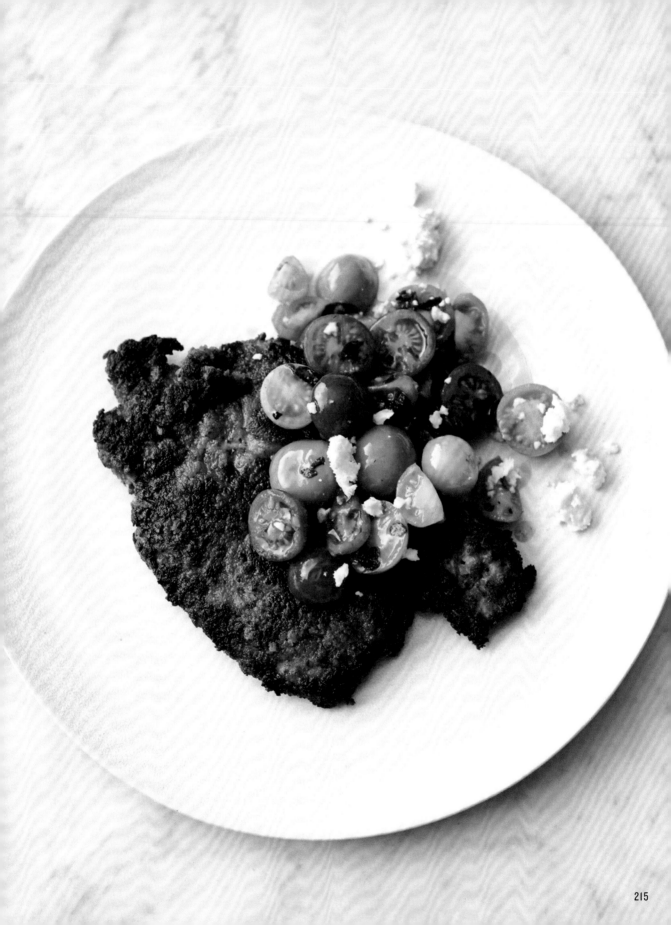

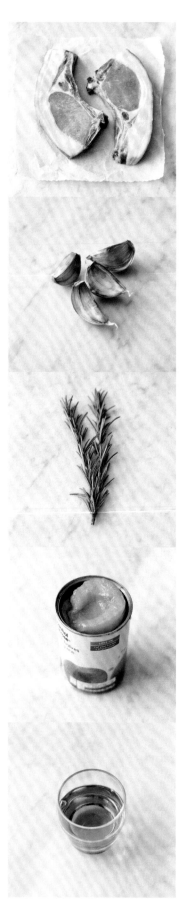

PEACHY PORK CHOPS

SERVES 2 | TOTAL 28 MINUTES

2 x 250g pork chops, with rind

4 cloves of garlic

2 sprigs of fresh rosemary

1 x 410g tin of peach halves in juice

50ml bourbon

Preheat the grill to high. Slice the rind off the chops, score the fat side of it in a criss-cross fashion and place skin side up in a tray. Pop under the grill for 5 minutes to crisp up into crackling – keep an eye on it. Season the chops with sea salt and black pepper, score the remaining fat in a criss-cross fashion, then sit the chops together fat edges down in a large cold non-stick frying pan. Place on a high heat for 3 to 4 minutes, or until golden and the fat has rendered out, using tongs to ensure they're in good contact with the pan. Gently turn the chops on to their sides to cook for 5 minutes on each side.

Meanwhile, peel and finely slice the garlic. Strip the rosemary leaves off the sprigs. Remove the chops to a plate, drain 90% of the fat from the pan into a jar to use for cooking another day, then sprinkle the garlic into the pan. Stir regularly until golden, then add the rosemary and four drained peach halves, flat side down. Jiggle over the heat until golden, then return the chops to the pan, add the bourbon and carefully set fire to it with a match (stand back!). Once the flames begin to subside, dish up with the crispy crackling.

CALORIES	FAT	SAT FAT	PROTEIN	CARBS	SUGAR	SALT	FIBRE
545kcal	32.1g	11.8g	29.4g	21.7g	20g	0.8g	0.1g

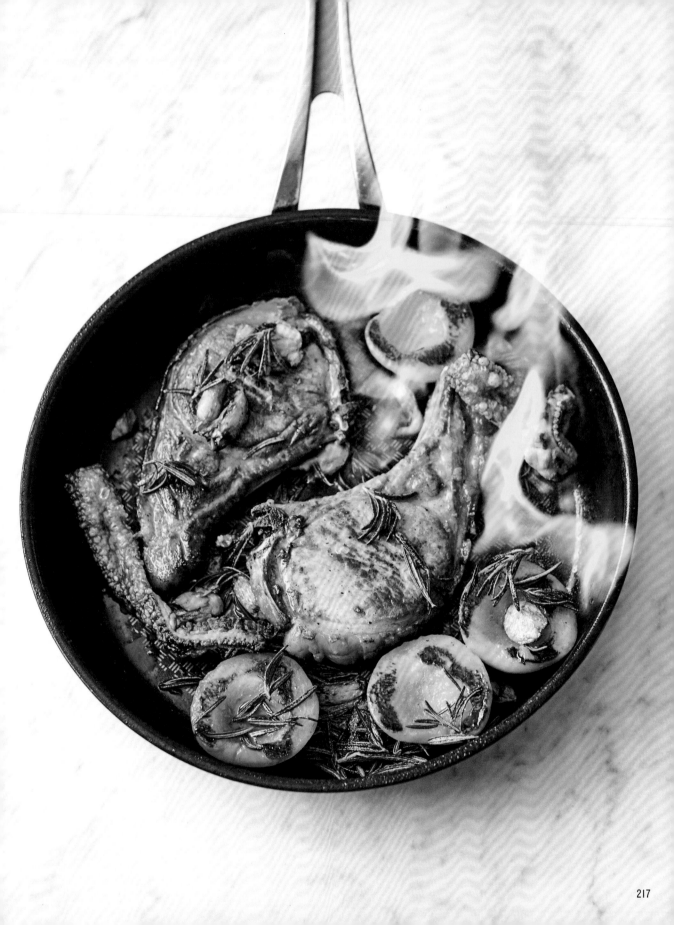

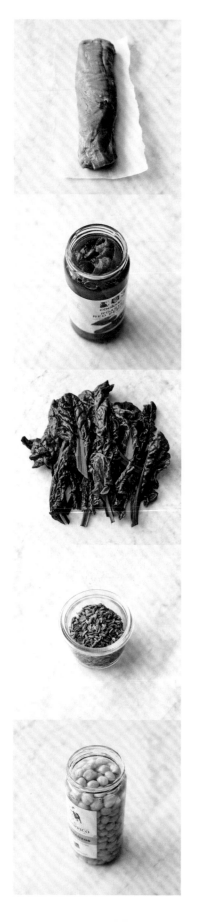

CHICKPEA CHARD PORK

SERVES 4 | TOTAL 29 MINUTES

400g piece of pork fillet

1 x 480g jar of roasted peeled peppers in brine

300g rainbow chard

1 heaped teaspoon fennel seeds

1 x 660g jar of chickpeas

Put a large shallow casserole pan on a high heat. Season the pork with sea salt and black pepper, then place in the pan with 1 tablespoon of olive oil and sear for 5 minutes, turning halfway. Meanwhile, drain the peppers and quickly dice into 1cm chunks, then trim and finely slice the chard, stalks and all.

Remove the pork to a plate, then add the fennel seeds, peppers and all the chard to the pork fat left behind in the pan. Stir and fry for 2 minutes, then pour in the chickpeas and their juice, stir, and bring to the boil. Sit the pork back in so it's touching the base of the pan, pour over any resting juices, cover, and simmer gently on a medium heat for 12 minutes, or until the pork is just cooked through and it all smells incredible, turning the pork occasionally.

Rest for 2 minutes, slice the pork, season the chickpeas to perfection, adding a splash of red wine vinegar, drizzle with extra virgin olive oil, and serve.

CALORIES	FAT	SAT FAT	PROTEIN	CARBS	SUGAR	SALT	FIBRE
325kcal	13.3g	3.4g	30.9g	20.9g	3.9g	1g	5.6g

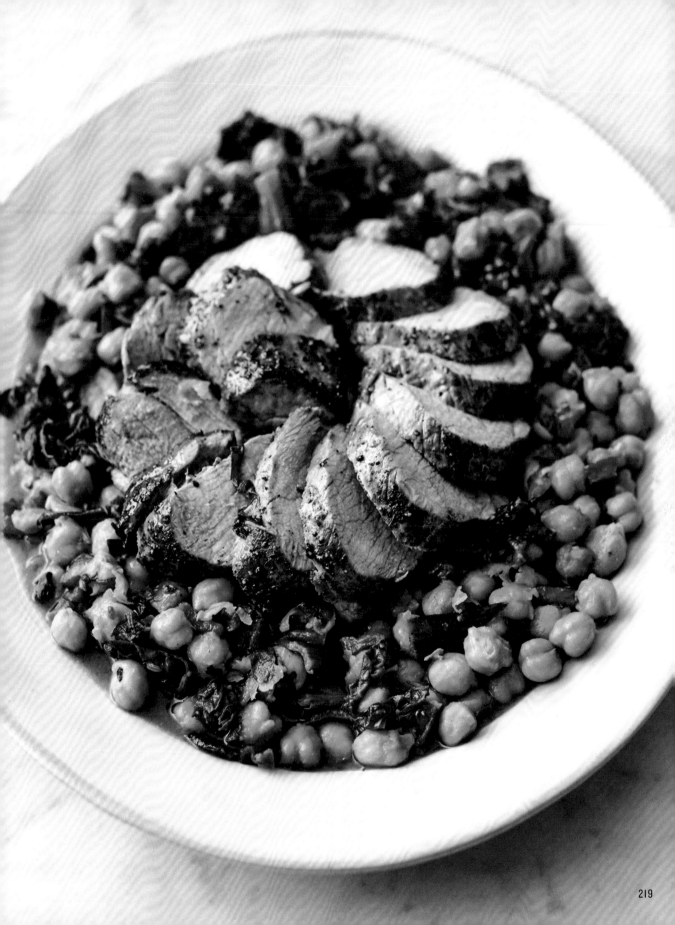

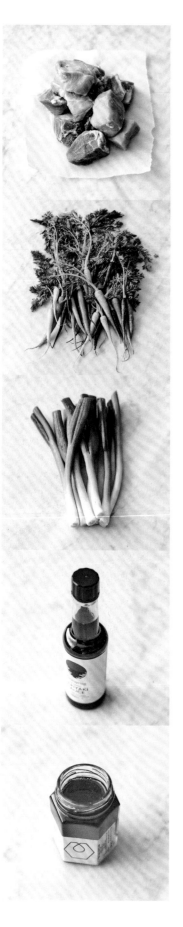

STICKY PORK STIR-FRY

SERVES 4 | TOTAL 18 MINUTES

400g pork shoulder

400g mixed-colour baby heritage carrots

8 spring onions

2 tablespoons teriyaki sauce

2 tablespoons runny honey

Put a large shallow casserole pan on a high heat. Chop the pork into 3cm chunks and place in the pan with 1 tablespoon of olive oil and a pinch of sea salt and black pepper. Trim and add the whole baby carrots (halving any larger ones), then cook for 12 minutes, or until everything is golden, tossing regularly. Meanwhile, trim and slice the spring onions.

Add a splash of water to the pan to deglaze it, then stir in the spring onions, teriyaki sauce and honey. Cook for another 3 minutes, tossing regularly until it's all shiny and sticky, then taste, season to perfection, and serve.

CALORIES	FAT	SAT FAT	PROTEIN	CARBS	SUGAR	SALT	FIBRE
332kcal	20g	5.9g	19.2g	20.1g	19g	1.3g	3.9g

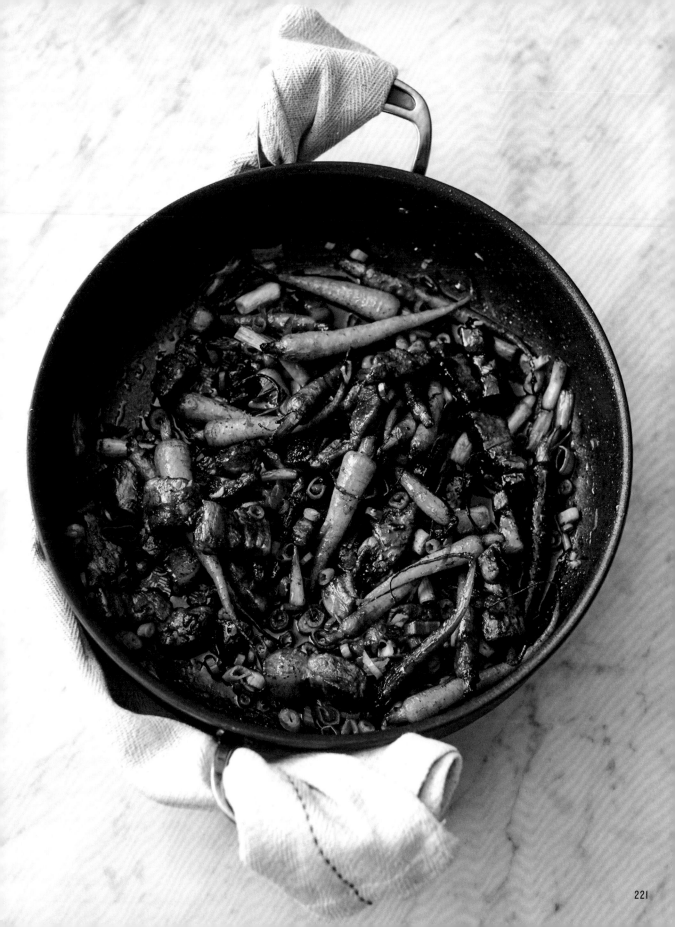

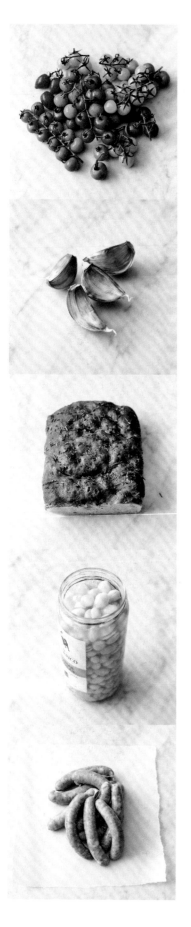

COMFORTING SAUSAGE BAKE

SERVES 4   FAST PREP 10 MINUTES   COOK 45 MINUTES

600g ripe mixed-colour cherry tomatoes

4 cloves of garlic

200g rosemary focaccia

1 x 660g jar of white beans

12 chipolatas

Preheat the oven to 180°C/350°F/gas 4. Halve the cherry tomatoes, peel and finely slice the garlic, and tear the bread into bite-sized chunks. Place it all in a 30cm x 35cm roasting tray, pour in the beans and their juice, drizzle with 1 tablespoon each of olive oil and red wine vinegar, add a splash of water, and mix it all together. Quickly pinch and twist each chipolata in the middle to make it into two mini ones, then randomly dot them around your bake, lightly pressing them into the beans and tomatoes.

Roast for 45 minutes, or until everything is golden, bubbling and delicious.

CALORIES	FAT	SAT FAT	PROTEIN	CARBS	SUGAR	SALT	FIBRE
571kcal	29g	8g	32.8g	43.8g	7g	1.6g	9.4g

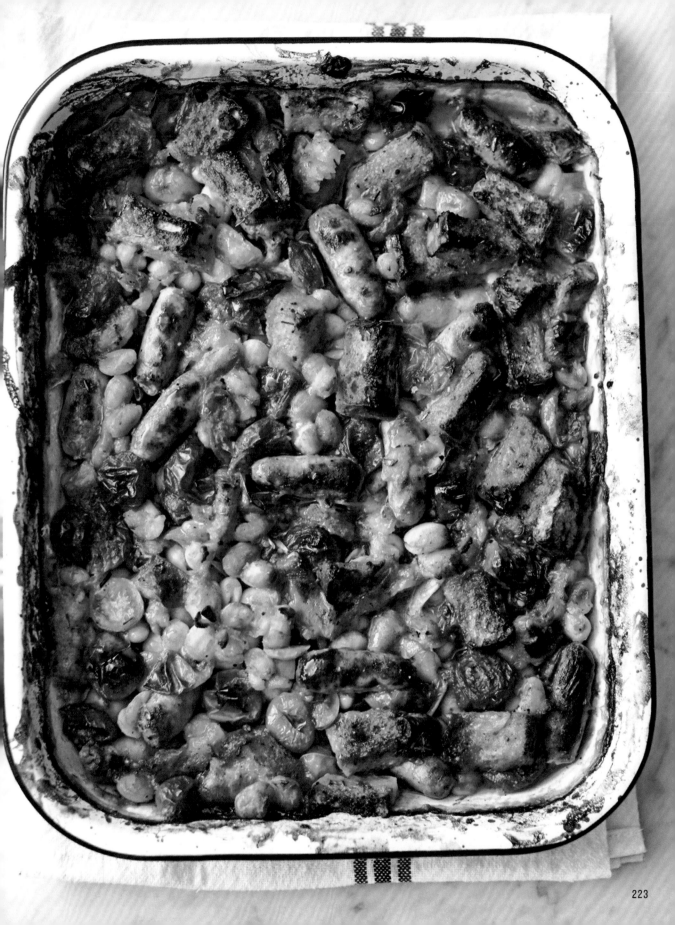

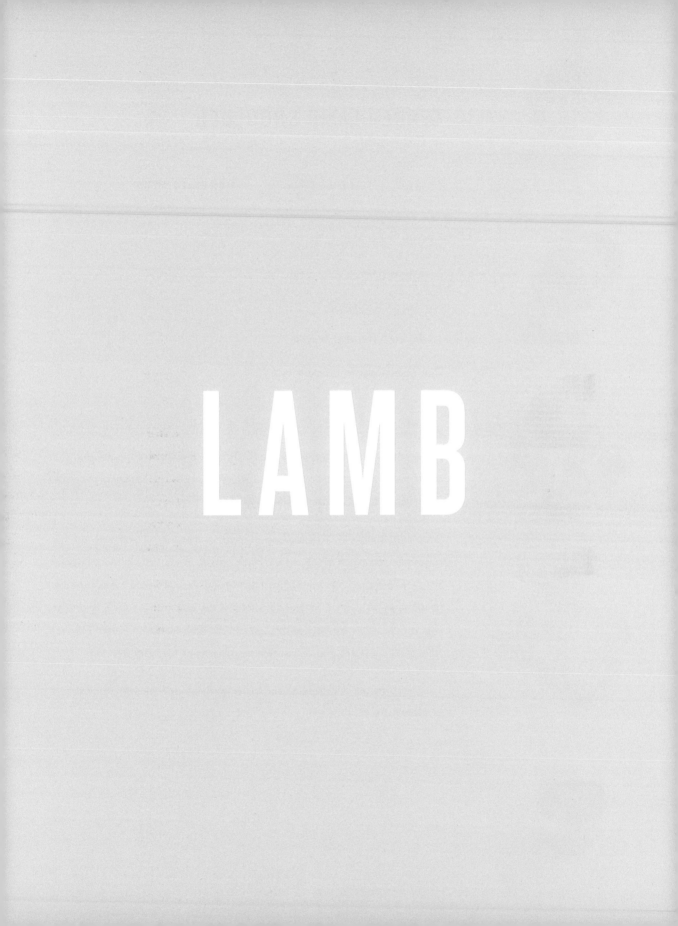
LAMB

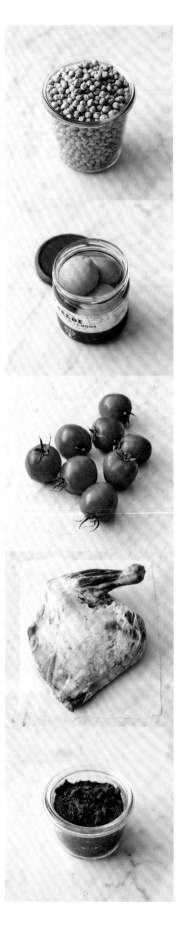

TENDER LAMB SHOULDER

SERVES 8   FAST PREP 10 MINUTES   SLOW COOK 6 HOURS

500g dried chickpeas

2 preserved lemons (20g each)

1kg ripe plum tomatoes

1 x 2kg lamb shoulder, bone in

2 heaped teaspoons ras el hanout

Pour the dried chickpeas into a 30cm x 40cm roasting tray. Quarter the preserved lemons and trim away the seedy core, then finely chop the rind and add to the tray with a good splash of liquor from their jar. Roughly chop the tomatoes, adding them to the tray as you go.

Drizzle the lamb with 1 tablespoon of olive oil, then rub all over with the ras el hanout and a pinch of sea salt and black pepper. Sit the lamb in the tray, pour in 1 litre of water, cover tightly with tin foil and place in a cold oven. Turn the temperature to 170°C/325°F/gas 3 and leave the lamb in there for 6 hours, or until the chickpeas are cooked through and the lamb is pullable – after 3 hours, stir a splash of water into the chickpeas, covering tightly again with foil.

To serve, taste the chickpeas, season to perfection, and drizzle with 1 tablespoon of extra virgin olive oil, then pull the lamb apart with two forks.

CALORIES	FAT	SAT FAT	PROTEIN	CARBS	SUGAR	SALT	FIBRE
522kcal	26.7g	10.2g	37.4g	35.3g	5.8g	0.7g	1.4g

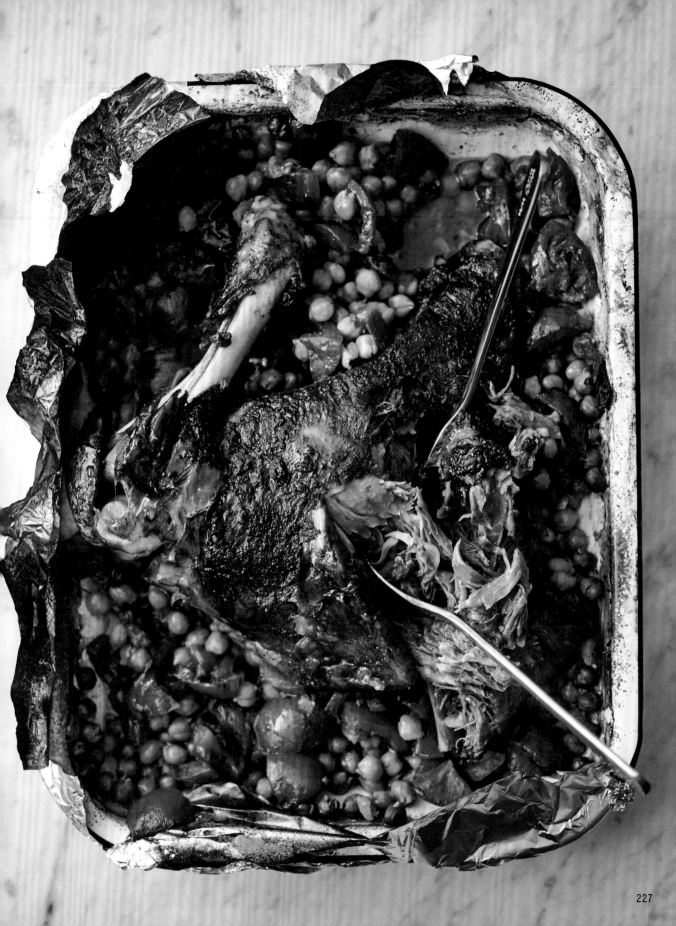

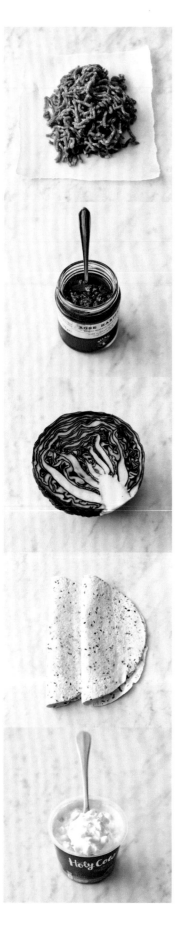

LAMB KOFTA FLATBREADS

SERVES 2   TOTAL JUST 15 MINUTES

250g minced lamb

2 teaspoons rose harissa, plus extra to serve

250g red cabbage

2 seeded wholemeal tortillas or flatbreads

2 tablespoons cottage cheese

Put a griddle pan on a high heat. Scrunch the minced lamb and harissa in your clean hands until well mixed. Divide into 6 pieces, then shape into koftas with your fingertips, leaving dents in the surface to increase the gnarly bits as they cook. Griddle for 4 to 5 minutes on each side, or until sizzling and golden.

Meanwhile, shred the red cabbage as finely as you can. Sprinkle with a pinch of sea salt and black pepper, drizzle with 1 tablespoon of red wine vinegar, then scrunch together to quickly pickle it.

Warm your tortillas or flatbreads, sprinkle over the cabbage, spoon over the cottage cheese, add the koftas, drizzle with a little extra harissa, and tuck in.

CALORIES	FAT	SAT FAT	PROTEIN	CARBS	SUGAR	SALT	FIBRE
451kcal	20g	8.9g	32.4g	32.7g	6.4g	1.3g	9g

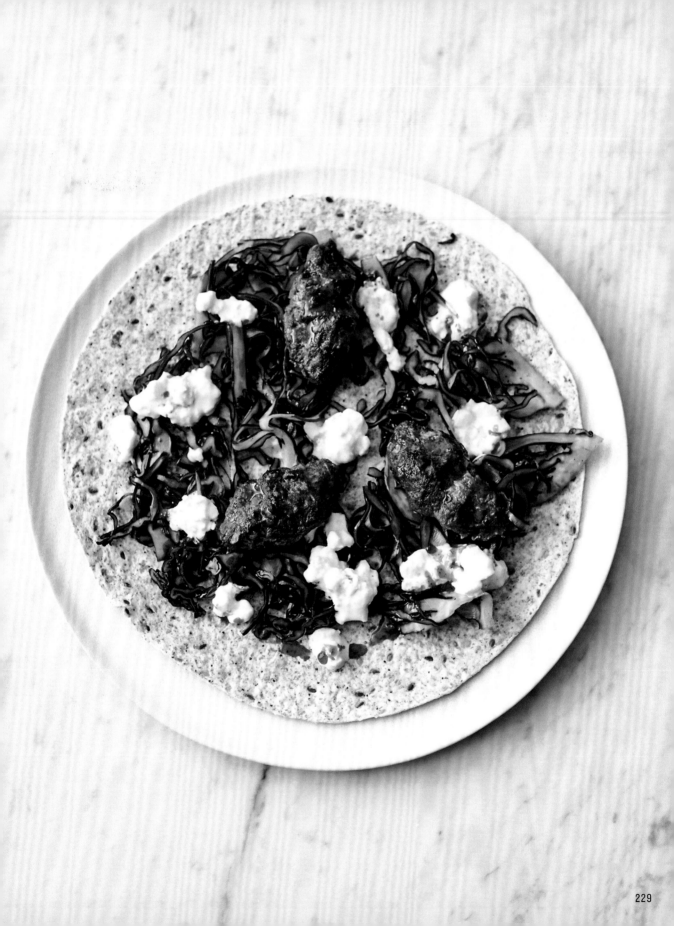

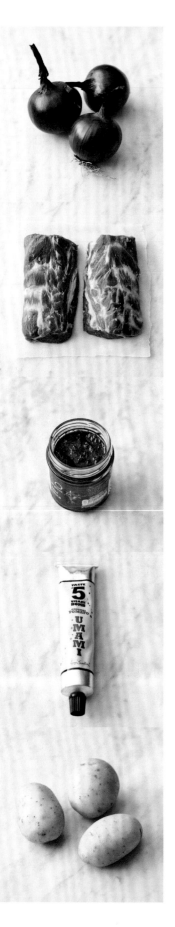

LOVELY LAMB HOTPOTS

SERVES 4   FAST PREP 10 MINUTES   SLOW COOK 2 HOURS

3 red onions

400g lamb neck fillet

6 teaspoons mint sauce

4 teaspoons umami paste

500g potatoes

Preheat the oven to 170°C/325°F/gas 3. Peel and roughly chop the onions, dice the lamb into 3cm chunks, then divide both between four 15cm ovenproof bowls, placing the bowls on a large oven tray. Add 1 teaspoon each of mint sauce and umami paste to each of the bowls, followed by 150ml of water and a little pinch of sea salt and black pepper. Stir well.

Quickly scrub the potatoes and rattle them through the thick slicer attachment of a food processor so they're just under ½cm thick. Divide between the bowls, overlapping them slightly to cover. Press down on the potato layer to compact everything, then cover with tin foil and bake for 2 hours, removing the foil for the last 30 minutes. Spoon over the remaining mint sauce, and tuck in.

CALORIES	FAT	SAT FAT	PROTEIN	CARBS	SUGAR	SALT	FIBRE
383kcal	18.4g	8.4g	22.6g	33.4g	10.4g	1.2g	4.4g

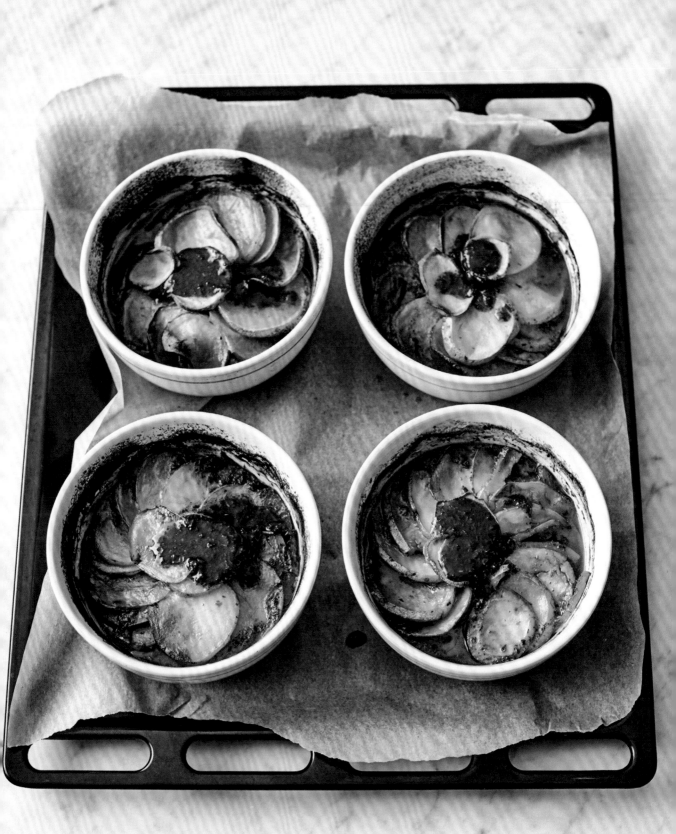

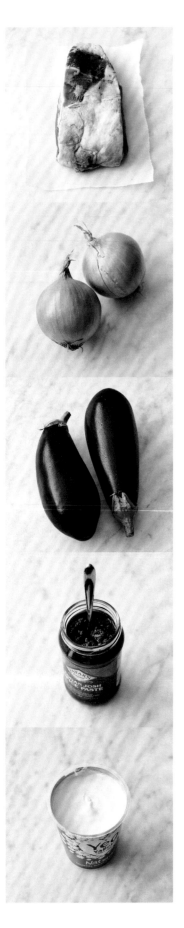

AROMATIC LAMB CURRY

SERVES 4 | FAST PREP 10 MINUTES | SLOW COOK 1 HOUR

400g lamb shoulder, bone out

2 large onions

2 large aubergines (800g total)

2 tablespoons rogan josh curry paste

200g natural yoghurt

Preheat the oven to 180°C/350°F/gas 4. Put a large shallow casserole pan on a high heat. Dice the lamb into 3cm chunks and place in the pan fat side down. Peel the onions, dice with the aubergines to the same size as the lamb, then stir into the pan. Season with sea salt and black pepper, stir in the curry paste and 1 tablespoon of red wine vinegar, then transfer to the oven for 1 hour, or until tender, stirring halfway and loosening with a splash of water, if needed.

Taste the curry, season to perfection, ripple through the yoghurt, drizzle over ½ a tablespoon of extra virgin olive oil, hit it with lots of black pepper, and serve.

CALORIES	FAT	SAT FAT	PROTEIN	CARBS	SUGAR	SALT	FIBRE
375kcal	24.8g	10.3g	23g	15.9g	13.5g	1.1g	2.6g

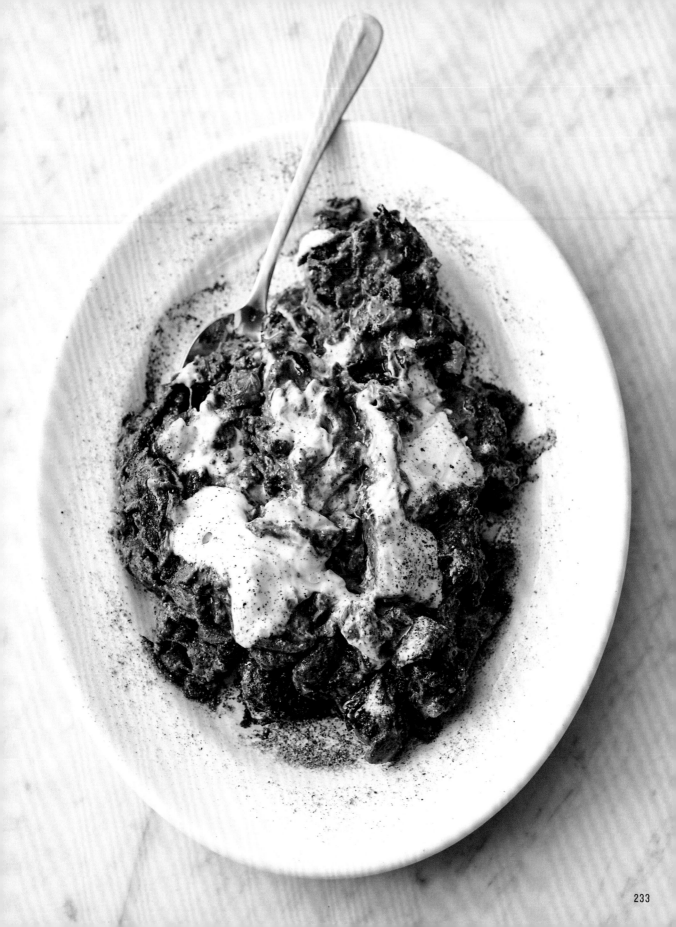

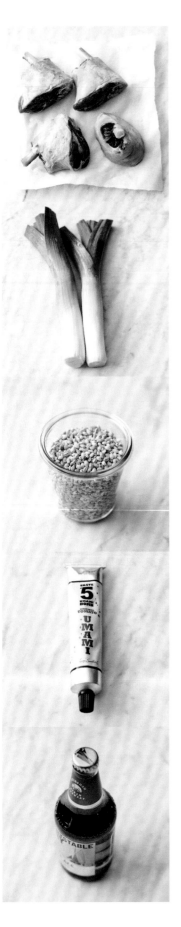

ALE BARLEY LAMB SHANKS

SERVES 4   FAST PREP 8 MINUTES   SLOW COOK 2 HOURS 30 MINUTES

4 lamb shanks (roughly 400g each)

2 leeks

200g pearl barley

I heaped tablespoon umami paste

500ml of your favourite ale

Preheat the oven to 170°C/325°F/gas 3. Place a large casserole pan on a high heat, and fry the lamb shanks in I tablespoon of olive oil, while you halve, wash and roughly chop the leeks. Add them to the pan with the pearl barley, umami paste and a pinch of sea salt and black pepper, then stir well. Pour in the ale and I tablespoon of red wine vinegar, then cover with 1.2 litres of water.

Cook in the oven for 2 hours 30 minutes, or until tender, then dish on up. Easy!

CALORIES	FAT	SAT FAT	PROTEIN	CARBS	SUGAR	SALT	FIBRE
783kcal	35.2g	12.8g	65.6g	48.8g	6.2g	1.5g	0.1g

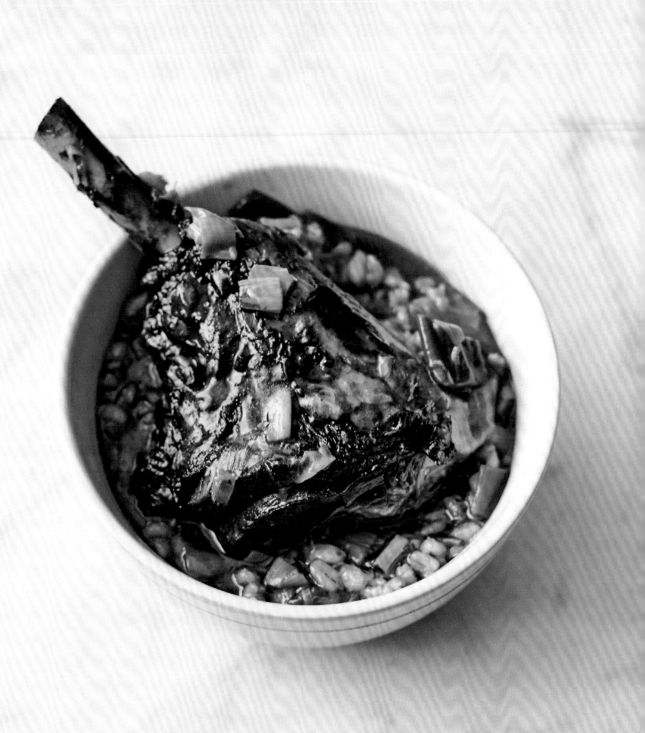

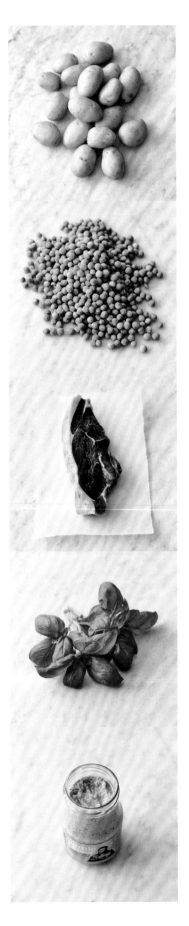

PAN-SEARED LAMB

SERVES 2   TOTAL 24 MINUTES

400g baby new potatoes

200g frozen peas

200g piece of lamb rump

4 sprigs of fresh basil

I heaped tablespoon yellow pepper or green pesto

Halve any larger potatoes, then cook in a pan of boiling salted water for 15 minutes, or until tender, adding the peas to the party for the last 3 minutes.

Meanwhile, rub the lamb all over with I teaspoon of olive oil, and a pinch of sea salt and black pepper. Starting fat side down, sear the lamb in a non-stick frying pan on a medium-high heat for 10 minutes, turning regularly until gnarly all over but blushing in the middle, or use your instincts to cook to your liking. Remove to a plate to rest, then, with the frying pan on a low heat, make a liquor by stirring in a splash of water and a little red wine vinegar to pick up all those nice sticky bits, leaving it to tick away slowly until needed.

Drain the potatoes and peas, tip into the liquor pan, pick over most of the basil, add the pesto and toss it all well. Serve with the lamb, sliced thinly, then pour over the resting juices. Pick over the remaining basil leaves, and tuck in.

CALORIES	FAT	SAT FAT	PROTEIN	CARBS	SUGAR	SALT	FIBRE
554kcal	24.5g	9.1g	40.4g	45.6g	4.9g	1.1g	7.8g

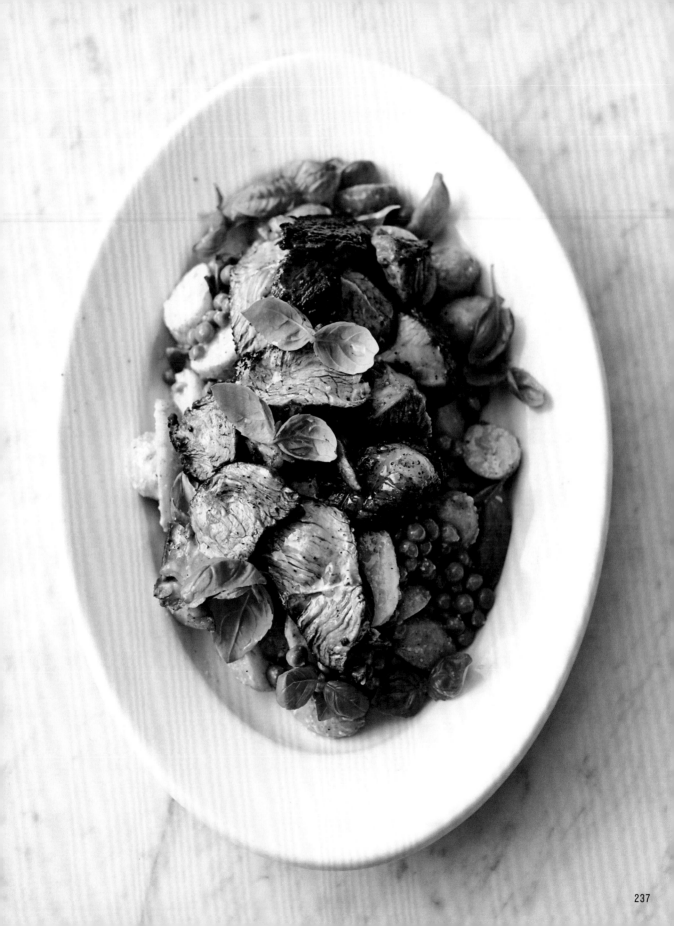

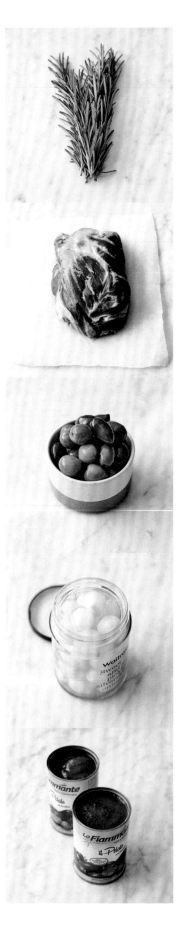

SUCCULENT LAMB STEW

SERVES 6 | FAST PREP 6 MINUTES | SLOW COOK 2 HOURS

½ a bunch of fresh rosemary (15g)

800g lamb shoulder, bone out

150g mixed-colour olives (stone in)

1 x 280g jar of silverskin pickled onions

2 x 400g tins of plum tomatoes

Preheat the oven to 170°C/325°F/gas 3. Place a 30cm shallow casserole pan on a high heat, strip in the rosemary leaves, add 1 tablespoon of olive oil, and crisp up for 1 minute while you dice the lamb into 3cm chunks. Scoop out the rosemary and put aside, adding the lamb to the pan for 2 minutes to get some colour. Meanwhile, squash the olives and remove the stones.

Drain the pickled onions and stir into the pan with the olives. Toss well, then pour in the tinned tomatoes, breaking them up with a wooden spoon, as well as 2 tins' worth of water. Cover and cook in the oven for 2 hours, or until thick, delicious and tender, stirring halfway and loosening with a splash of water, if needed. Taste, season to perfection with sea salt and black pepper, sprinkle over the crispy rosemary leaves, and serve. Simple.

CALORIES	FAT	SAT FAT	PROTEIN	CARBS	SUGAR	SALT	FIBRE
398kcal	29.6g	12.2g	25.6g	7.6g	6.8g	1.6g	2.2g

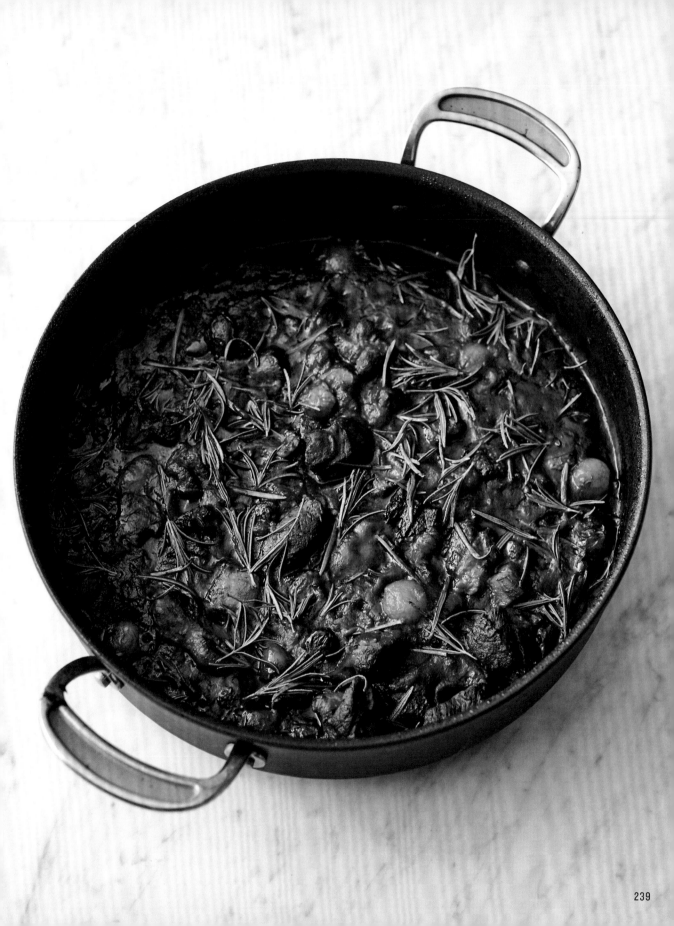

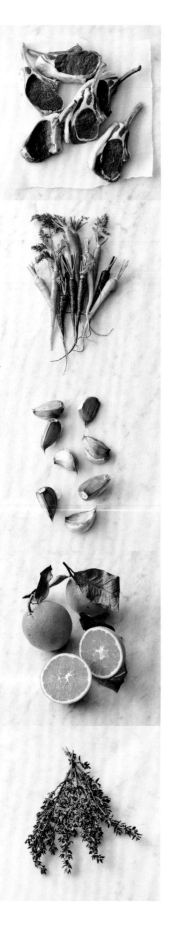

STICKY LAMB CHOPS

SERVES 2 | TOTAL JUST 15 MINUTES

6 lamb chops, French-trimmed (600g total)

200g mixed-colour baby heritage carrots

8 cloves of garlic

3 oranges

½ a bunch of fresh thyme (15g)

Score the fat of the lamb chops, season them with sea salt and black pepper, then line them up, like a rack, and sit them together fat edges down in a large shallow casserole pan on a medium-high heat. Leave for 5 minutes to render and crisp up. Trim and add the whole baby carrots (halving any larger ones) and the unpeeled garlic cloves alongside, turning the carrots regularly.

Gently turn the chops on to their sides, to cook for 2 minutes on each side, or until golden, but still pink in the middle. Meanwhile, use a speed-peeler to peel strips of zest from 1 orange. Sprinkle them into the pan with the thyme sprigs, and toss it all together for just 30 seconds to get the flavours going.

Remove the chops to a plate to rest, then squeeze the juice from all 3 oranges into the pan. Let the juice bubble and reduce until sticky, quickly toss the lamb back in with its resting juices, then hey presto, time to dish up.

CALORIES	FAT	SAT FAT	PROTEIN	CARBS	SUGAR	SALT	FIBRE
571kcal	36.2g	14.7g	26.5g	36.7g	32.1g	0.8g	8.5g

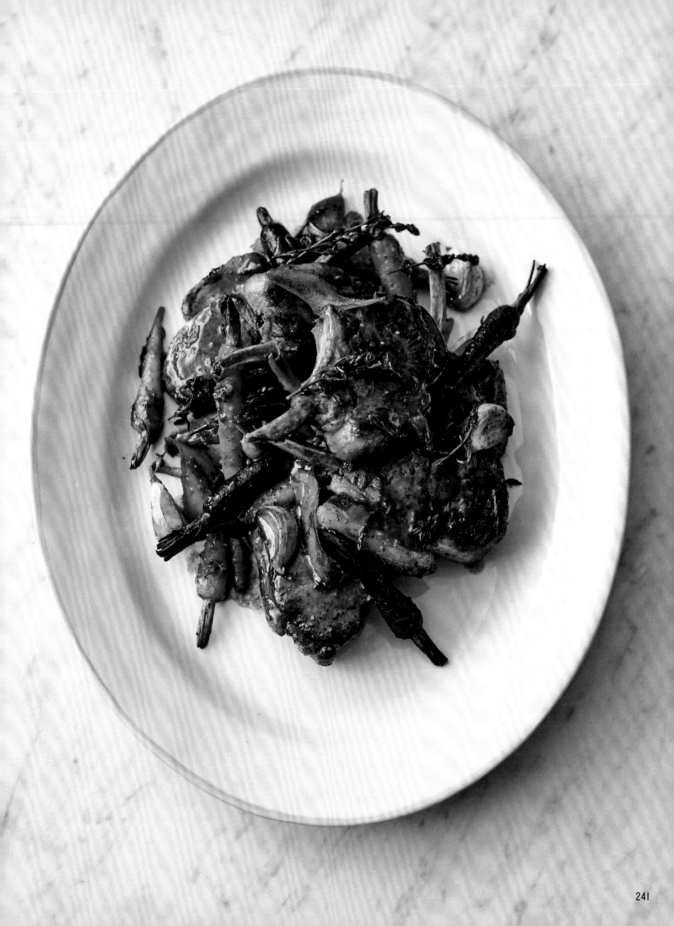

RICE & NOODLES

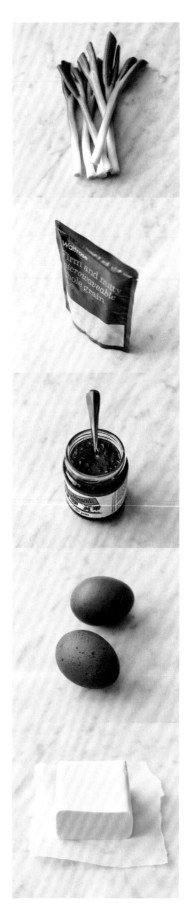

EGG-FRIED RICE

SERVES 2 | TOTAL JUST 10 MINUTES

6 spring onions

1 x 250g sachet of cooked brown basmati rice

2 heaped teaspoons chilli jam

2 large eggs

150g firm silken tofu

Put a large non-stick frying pan on a medium-high heat. Trim and finely slice the spring onions and fry with 1 tablespoon of olive oil for 1 minute. Add the rice, chilli jam, a splash of water and a pinch of sea salt and black pepper, then toss for 2 minutes until everything is well coated.

Push the rice to the sides of the pan, making a big well in the middle. Crack the eggs into the well, then use a rubber spatula to start gently moving the eggs around to create big curds. Break in the tofu, then fold the rice back through the egg until it's all looking good. Taste and season to perfection. Lightly oil the inside of a bowl, add the egg-fried rice, gently compacting it with the spatula, then proudly turn out on to a plate, retro style.

CALORIES	FAT	SAT FAT	PROTEIN	CARBS	SUGAR	SALT	FIBRE
395kcal	17.1g	3.6g	18.2g	44.8g	8.1g	0.7g	2.1g

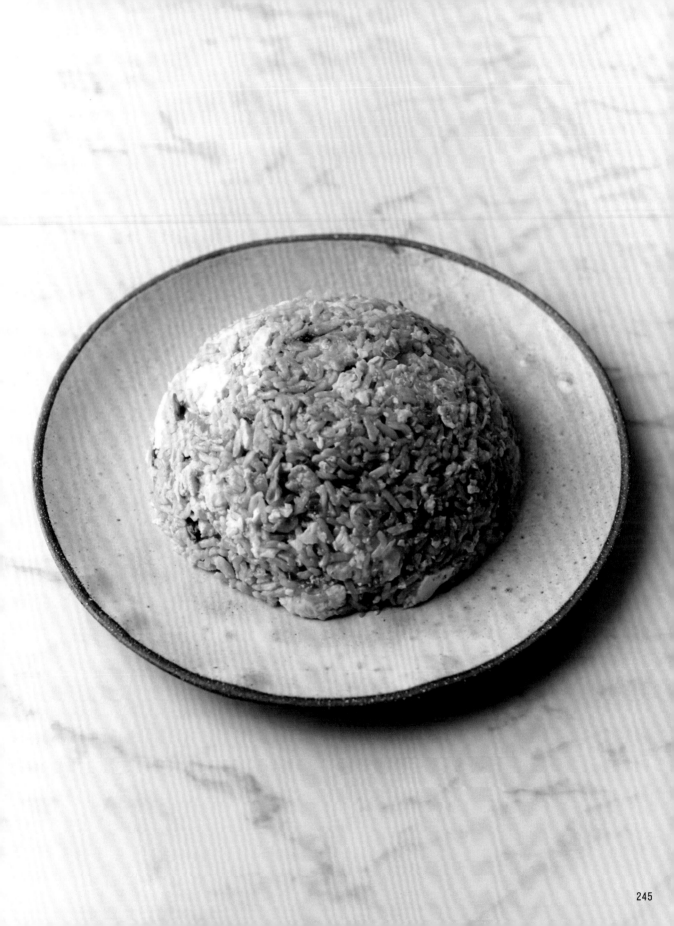

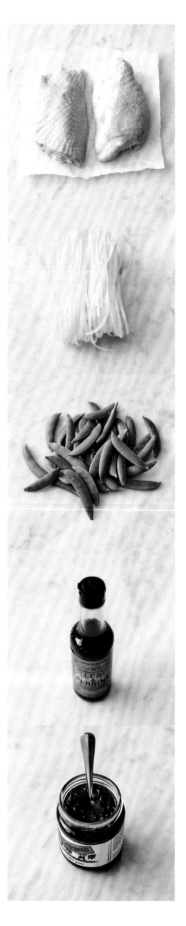

SWEET & SOUR CHICKEN NOODLES

SERVES 2   TOTAL 20 MINUTES

2 x 200g chicken thighs, skin on, bone in

150g fine rice noodles

200g sugar snap peas

2 tablespoons Worcestershire sauce

2 teaspoons chilli jam

Pull the skin off the chicken. Place the skin in a large non-stick frying pan on a medium heat to render and get golden, turning occasionally. Cut the bones out of the thighs and chuck into the pan for bonus flavour, then chop the meat into 2cm pieces. Move the skin and bones to one side of the pan, then add the meat alongside and cook for 5 minutes, or until golden, stirring occasionally. Once crispy, remove, chop and reserve the skin, discarding the bones.

Meanwhile, cook the noodles in boiling salted water according to the packet instructions. Halve the sugar snaps lengthways. Once soft, drain the noodles, reserving a mugful of cooking water, then refresh under cold water. Use scissors to snip the noodles into roughly 8cm lengths.

Stir the Worcestershire sauce and chilli jam into the chicken pan and let the jam melt, then add the sugar snaps and noodles. Toss over the heat for 2 minutes, adding a splash of reserved noodle water to loosen, if needed. Taste and season to perfection with sea salt and black pepper, then dish up and sprinkle over the reserved crispy chicken skin.

CALORIES	FAT	SAT FAT	PROTEIN	CARBS	SUGAR	SALT	FIBRE
544kcal	14.7g	4.1g	26.2g	74.8g	12.2g	0.7g	1.7g

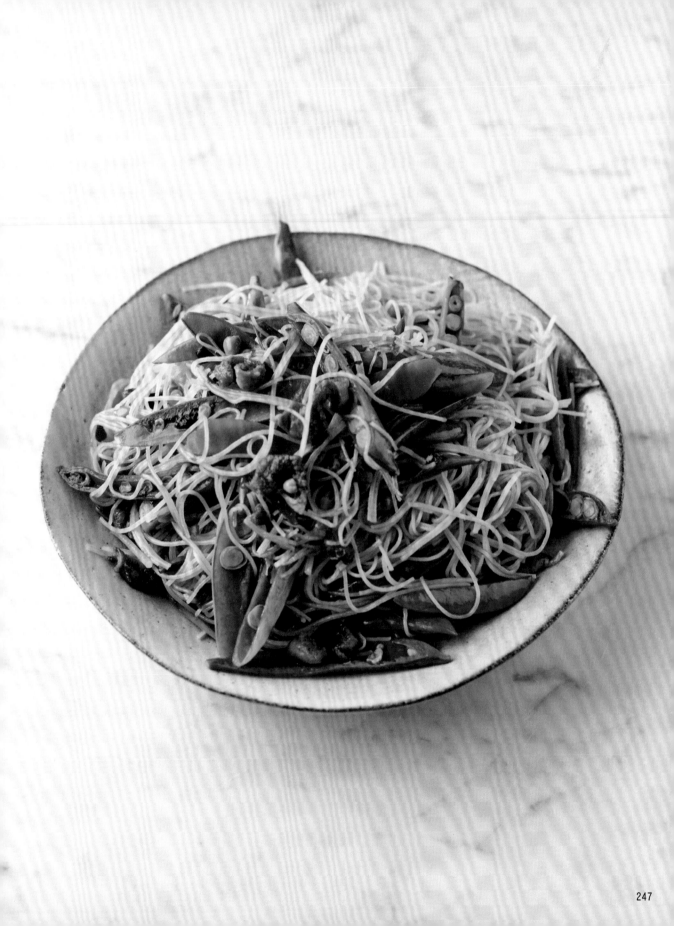

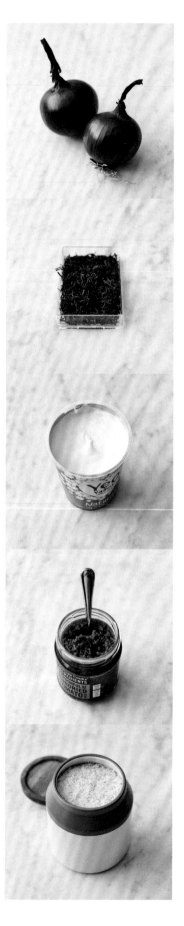

BAKED SAFFRON RICE

SERVES 4 | TOTAL 26 MINUTES

2 red onions

2 small pinches of saffron

4 heaped tablespoons natural yoghurt

4 tablespoons sun-dried tomato paste

300g white basmati rice

Preheat the oven to 200°C/400°F/gas 6. Peel and finely chop the red onions. Place a 25cm x 30cm roasting tray on a high heat on the hob, pour in 1 tablespoon of olive oil, add the onions and fry for 4 minutes, or until soft and sweet, stirring regularly. Meanwhile, place half the saffron in 600ml of boiling kettle water. In a bowl, cover the remaining saffron with 1 tablespoon of boiling water, steep for 10 seconds, then mix with the yoghurt and put aside.

Stir the tomato paste, rice and a pinch of sea salt and black pepper into the onion tray, then pour in the saffron water and bring to the boil. Once boiling, carefully transfer to the oven for 15 minutes, or until the rice has absorbed all the liquid, fluffed up beautifully and is golden and crisp on top.

Spoon the saffron yoghurt over the rice, drizzle it all with 1 tablespoon of extra virgin olive oil, fork and mix it all together, and dish up.

CALORIES	FAT	SAT FAT	PROTEIN	CARBS	SUGAR	SALT	FIBRE
506kcal	20.1g	3.6g	9.7g	74.9g	10.5g	1.2g	4.1g

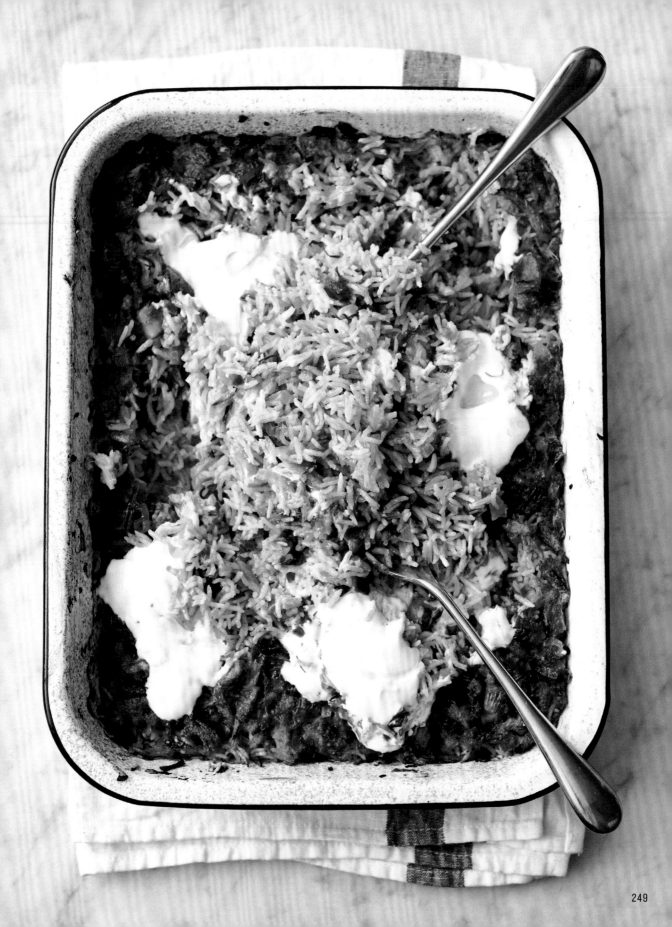

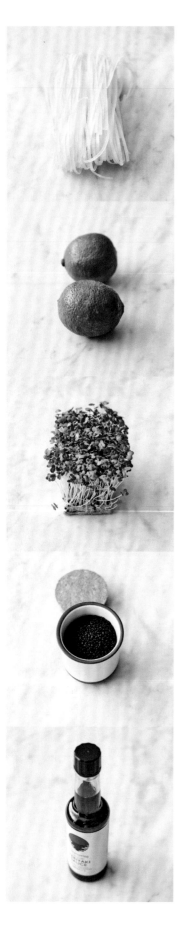

BLACK TAHINI NOODLES

SERVES 2 | TOTAL JUST 13 MINUTES

150g fine rice noodles

2 limes

1 punnet of cress

50g black sesame seeds

2 tablespoons teriyaki sauce

Cook the noodles in boiling salted water according to the packet instructions, then drain, reserving a mugful of cooking water. Meanwhile, finely grate the zest of 1 lime, snip the cress and put both aside. Toast the sesame seeds in a dry non-stick frying pan on a high heat for 1 minute, tossing regularly. Reserving one quarter of the seeds, pound the rest in a pestle and mortar until fairly fine, then muddle in the teriyaki and the juice of 1 lime. Taste, season to perfection with sea salt and black pepper, and you've got a black tahini!

Toss the noodles and black tahini together, loosening with a splash of reserved noodle water. Serve sprinkled with the lime zest, cress and reserved seeds, with lime wedges on the side, for squeezing over.

CALORIES	FAT	SAT FAT	PROTEIN	CARBS	SUGAR	SALT	FIBRE
453kcal	14.7g	2.6g	8.9g	68.5g	6.1g	1.2g	2.2g

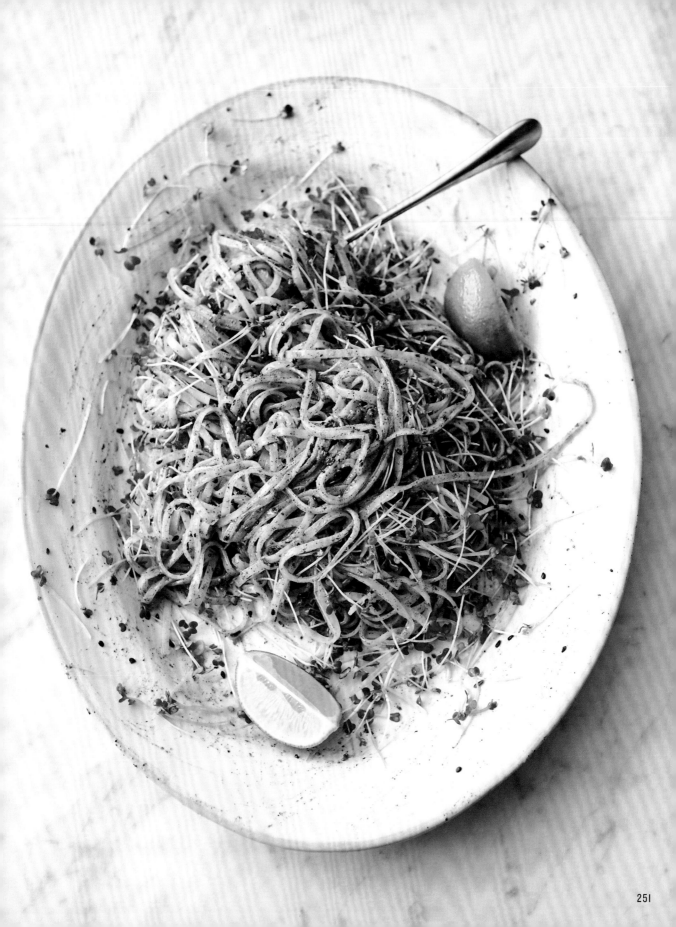

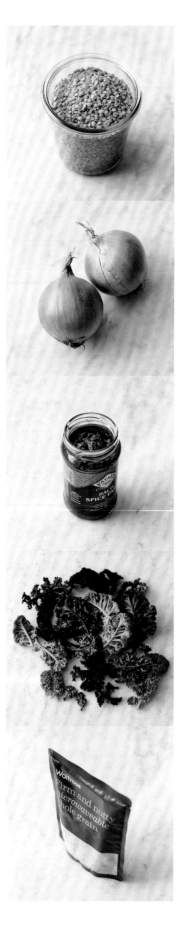

SPICED LENTILS & RICE

SERVES 2-4 | TOTAL 25 MINUTES

75g dried red split lentils

2 onions

2 heaped tablespoons balti curry paste

200g mixed-colour kale

1 x 250g sachet of cooked brown basmati rice

Cook the lentils in a pan of boiling salted water according to the packet instructions. Meanwhile, peel and finely slice the onions, put them into a large shallow casserole pan on a medium heat with ½ a tablespoon of olive oil and the balti paste, and cook for 15 minutes, or until soft and golden, stirring regularly. Tear in the kale (discarding any tough stalks), add a splash of lentil cooking water, cover and leave for 2 minutes.

Drain the lentils, toss into the casserole pan with the rice, cover again, and leave for a final 3 minutes. Toss it all together, taste, season to perfection with sea salt and black pepper, and dish up. Delicious.

CALORIES	FAT	SAT FAT	PROTEIN	CARBS	SUGAR	SALT	FIBRE
502kcal	14.8g	1g	19.9g	76.9g	16.3g	1.5g	7.9g

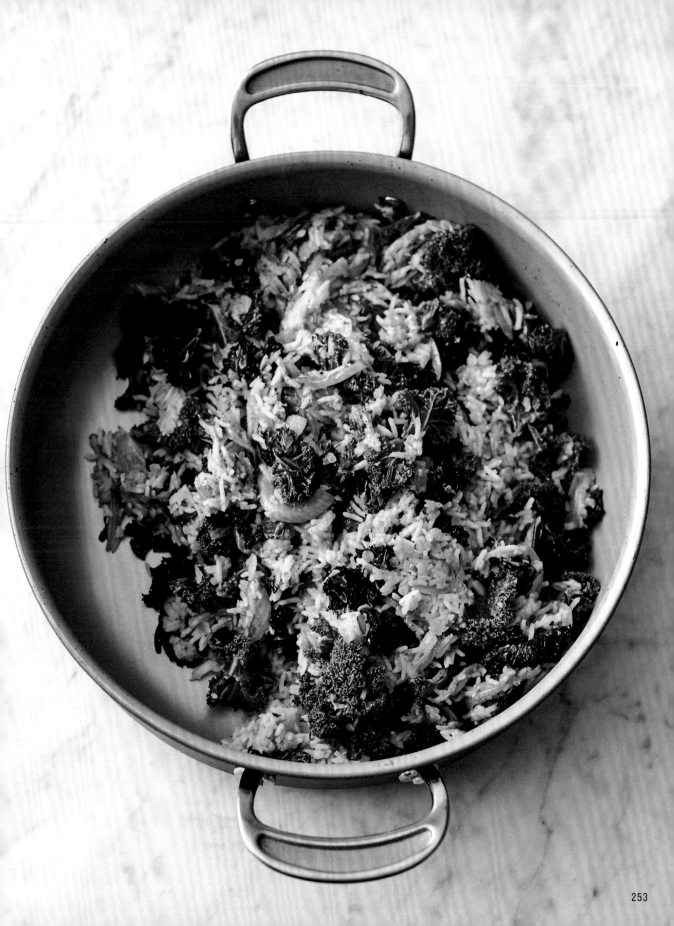

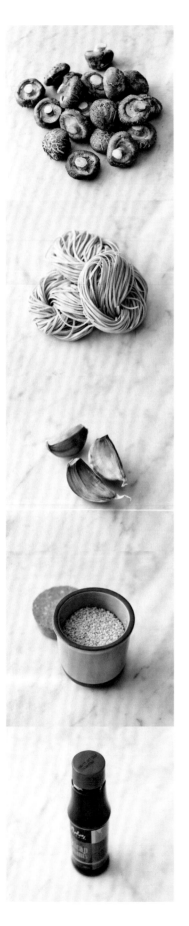

SESAME SHIITAKE EGG NOODLES

SERVES 2 | TOTAL JUST 13 MINUTES

400g shiitake mushrooms

150g egg noodles

3 cloves of garlic

3 tablespoons sesame seeds

3 tablespoons kicap manis

Halve the mushrooms, then dry toast in a large non-stick frying pan on a medium-high heat for 8 minutes, or until golden and nutty, tossing occasionally. Meanwhile, cook the noodles in a pan of boiling salted water according to the packet instructions, then drain, reserving a mugful of cooking water. Peel and finely slice the garlic, add to the mushroom pan with 1 tablespoon of olive oil and cook for a further 2 minutes, tossing regularly.

Pound the sesame seeds until fine in a pestle and mortar, then toss into the pan with the noodles, kicap manis and a good splash of reserved noodle water until everything is well coated. Taste, season to perfection with sea salt and black pepper, if needed, and dish right up.

CALORIES	FAT	SAT FAT	PROTEIN	CARBS	SUGAR	SALT	FIBRE
562kcal	17.3g	3g	15.8g	90.5g	11g	1.5g	0.6g

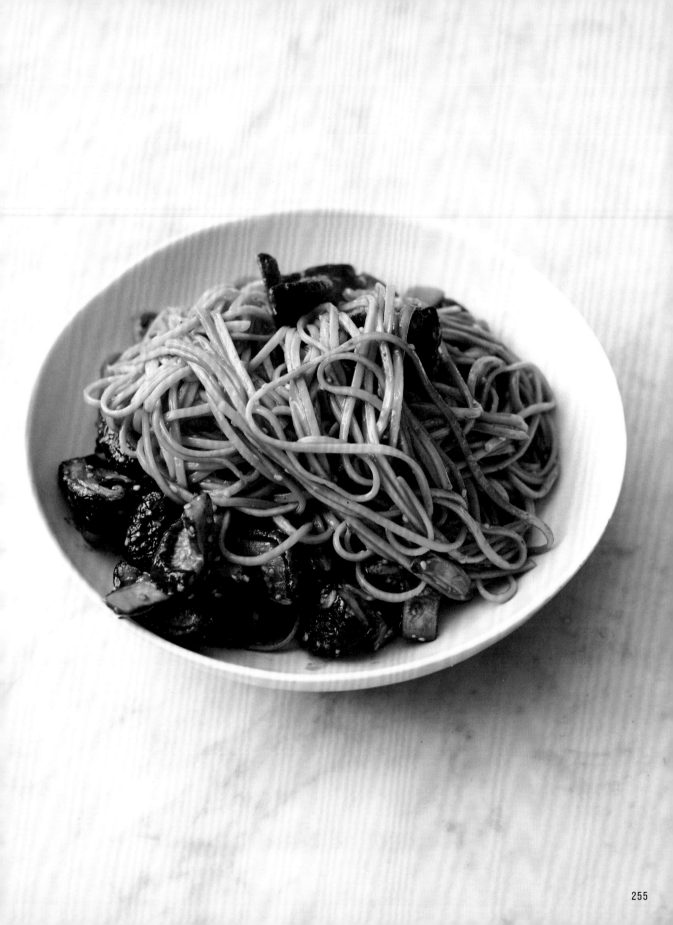

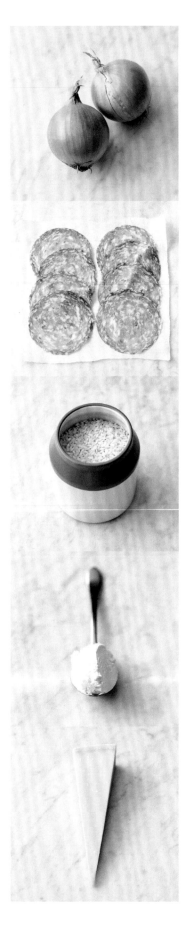

ITALIAN BAKED RICE

SERVES 4 | FAST PREP 10 MINUTES | COOK 40 MINUTES

2 onions

60g fennel salami

300g Arborio risotto rice

1 heaped tablespoon mascarpone cheese

40g Parmesan cheese

Preheat the oven to 180°C/350°F/gas 4. Place a large shallow casserole pan on a high heat. Peel and quarter the onions and quickly break apart into petals straight into the pan. Char for 4 minutes, tossing regularly. Reduce to a medium heat and stir in 1 tablespoon of olive oil and the salami, then the rice, followed 1 minute later by 1.2 litres of boiling kettle water and the mascarpone. Finely grate and stir in the Parmesan with a pinch of sea salt and black pepper.

Transfer the pan to the oven for 40 minutes, or until the rice has absorbed all the liquid and is just cooked through. Drizzle with 1 tablespoon of extra virgin olive oil and dish up, seasoning to perfection at the table.

CALORIES	FAT	SAT FAT	PROTEIN	CARBS	SUGAR	SALT	FIBRE
503kcal	20.2g	8g	13g	71.7g	6.3g	1.2g	3g

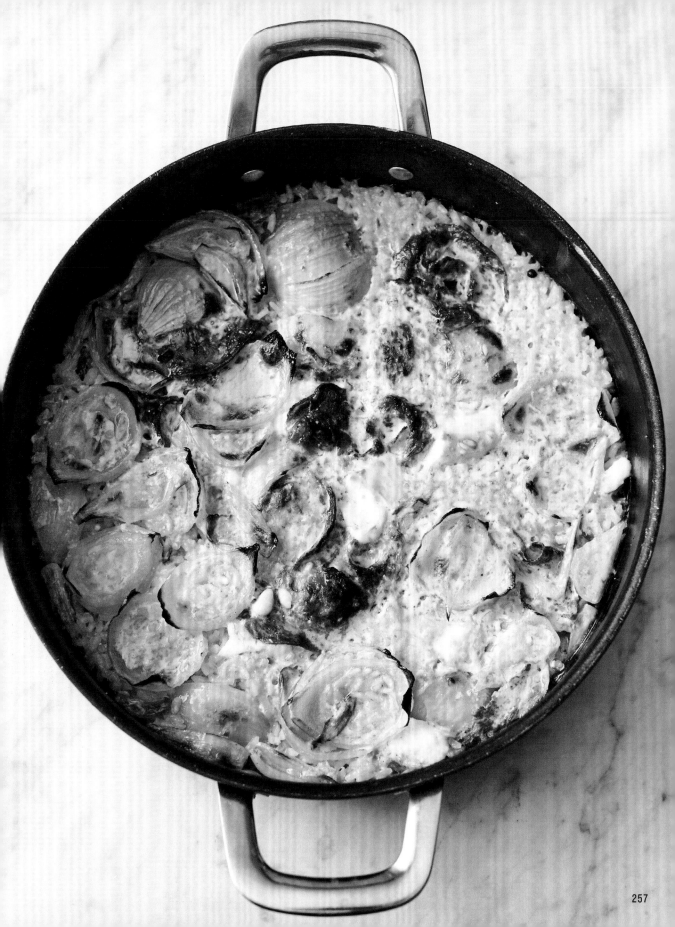

257

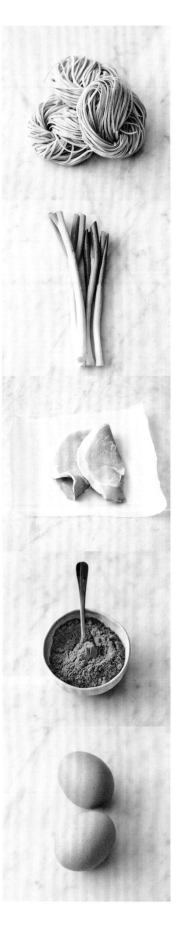

HAM & EGG CURRIED NOODLES

SERVES 2 | TOTAL JUST 10 MINUTES

150g egg noodles

4 spring onions

100g roast ham

2 teaspoons curry powder

2 large eggs

Cook the noodles in a pan of boiling salted water according to the packet instructions, then drain, reserving a mugful of cooking water. Meanwhile, trim and finely slice the spring onions, and finely slice the ham.

Place the ham in a non-stick frying pan on a medium-high heat with 1 tablespoon of olive oil and the curry powder. While it gets nicely golden, beat the eggs. Pour them into the pan, moving them around with a rubber spatula until they start to cook, then stir in the noodles and most of the spring onions. Toss over the heat for 2 minutes, then taste and season to perfection with sea salt and black pepper, loosening with a splash of reserved noodle water, if needed. Dish up the noodles, scatter over the remaining spring onions and finish with 1 teaspoon of extra virgin olive oil.

CALORIES	FAT	SAT FAT	PROTEIN	CARBS	SUGAR	SALT	FIBRE
561kcal	26.7g	5.8g	28.4g	55.8g	1.8g	2.7g	0.6g

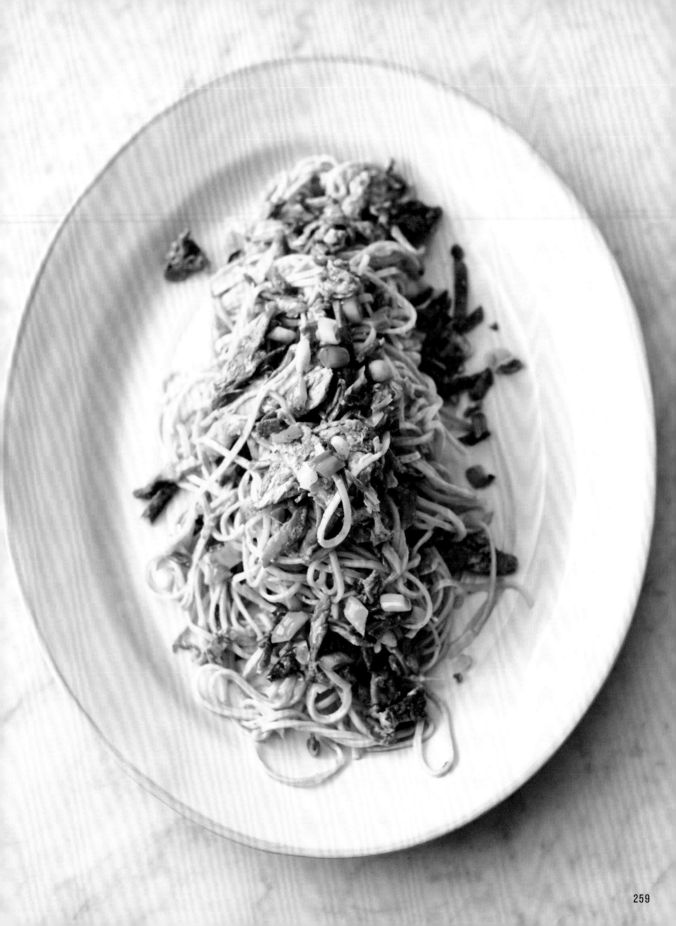

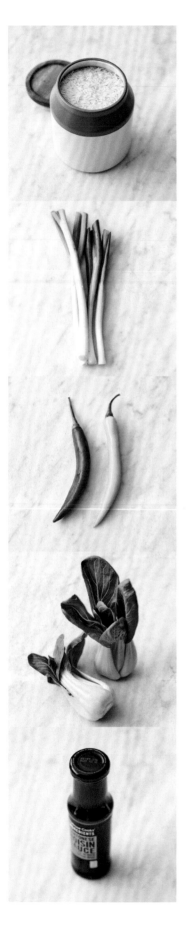

HOISIN PAK CHOI RICE

SERVES 2 | TOTAL JUST 15 MINUTES

150g white basmati rice

4 spring onions

2 fresh mixed-colour chillies

2 pak choi (250g)

2 tablespoons hoisin sauce

Cook the rice in a pan of boiling salted water according to the packet instructions, then drain. Meanwhile, trim and finely slice the spring onions, putting the white slices into a bowl. Deseed and finely chop the chillies, add to the bowl with 1 tablespoon of red wine vinegar and a little sea salt and black pepper, and mix well to make a dressing.

Halve the pak choi lengthways and place in a large non-stick frying pan on a medium-high heat with 1 tablespoon of olive oil. Once charred, toss in the green spring onion slices, then stir in the hoisin. Let it glaze for 1 minute, then mix in the rice for 1 final minute. Spoon over the chilli dressing, and serve up.

CALORIES	FAT	SAT FAT	PROTEIN	CARBS	SUGAR	SALT	FIBRE
378kcal	7.3g	1.1g	8.5g	73.3g	9.3g	1g	2.9g

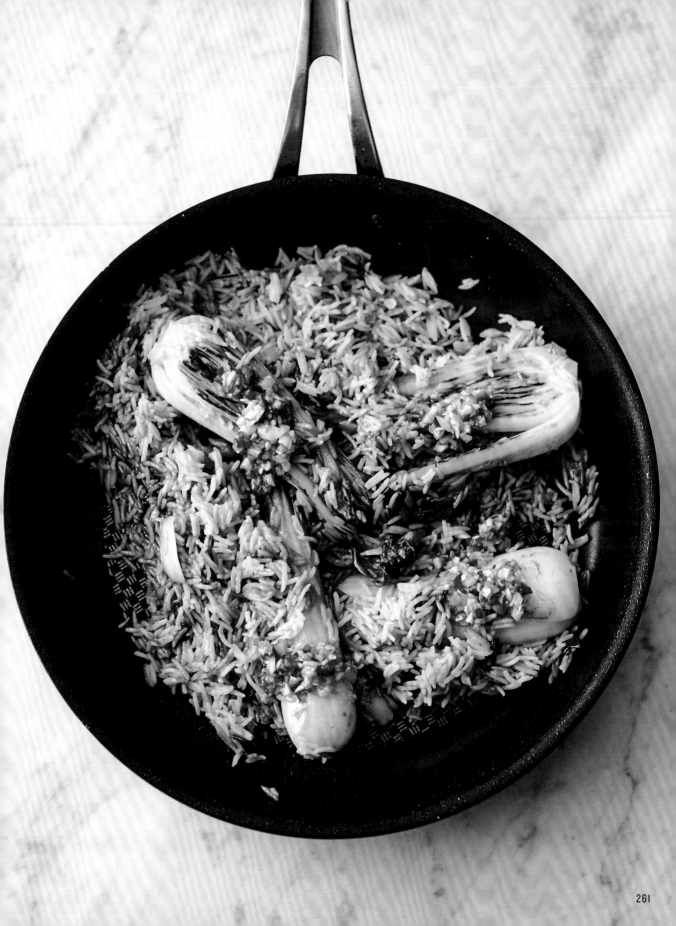

SWEET TREATS

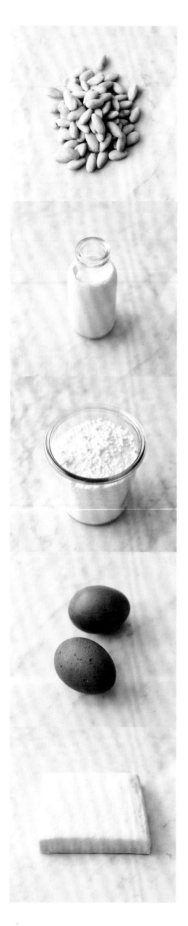

ALMOND PASTRY PUFF

SERVES 6   TOTAL 28 MINUTES

100g blanched almonds

1 tablespoon double cream, plus extra to serve

75g icing sugar, plus extra for dusting

2 large eggs

375g block of all-butter puff pastry (cold)

Preheat the oven to 220°C/425°F/gas 7. Line a baking tray with greaseproof paper. Blitz the almonds in a food processor until nice and fine. With the processor still running, add the cream, icing sugar, 1 egg and a pinch of sea salt until combined, stopping to scrape down the sides with a spatula, if needed.

Halve the pastry, shape into two rounds and, working quickly, dusting with icing sugar as you go to stop the pastry sticking, roll out between two sheets of greaseproof paper until they're just under ½cm thick. Place one round on the lined tray. Spread the almond paste on top, leaving a 2cm gap at the edges. Put the other round on top and gently push together. Quickly seal the edges with the back of a fork. Eggwash the top, then dust over an extra layer of sugar.

Gently push your finger into the middle of the pastry, then, with a sharp knife, very delicately make little lines from the centre to the outside. Bake on the bottom of the oven for 12 to 15 minutes, or until puffed up and golden, dusting with a little extra icing sugar before dishing up.

CALORIES	FAT	SAT FAT	PROTEIN	CARBS	SUGAR	SALT	FIBRE
443kcal	29.2g	12.7g	8.9g	36.7g	14.7g	0.7g	0.9g

SWEET TREATS

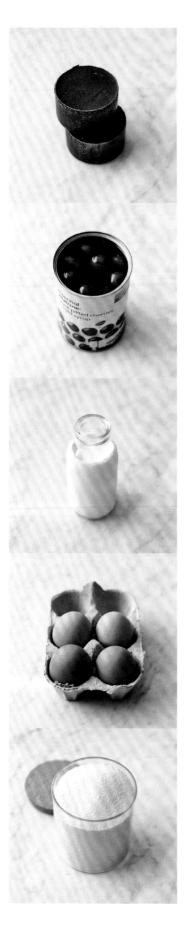

CHERRY CHOCOLATE MOUSSE

SERVES 6   TOTAL 30 MINUTES

200g dark chocolate (70%)

1 x 400g tin of black pitted cherries in syrup

200ml double cream

4 large eggs

2 tablespoons golden caster sugar

Melt the chocolate in a heatproof bowl over a pan of gently simmering water, then remove to cool for 10 minutes. Meanwhile, simmer the cherries and their syrup in a non-stick frying pan on a medium heat until thick, then remove.

Whip the cream to very soft peaks. Separate the eggs, add the yolks to the cream with the sugar, and whisk to combine. Add a pinch of sea salt to the whites and, with a clean whisk, beat until super-stiff. Fold the cooled chocolate into the cream, then very gently fold that through the egg whites with a spatula.

Divvy up the mousse between six glasses or bowls, interspersing the cherries and syrup throughout, and finishing with a few nice cherries on top.

CALORIES	FAT	SAT FAT	PROTEIN	CARBS	SUGAR	SALT	FIBRE
406kcal	25.4g	14.8g	7.6g	40g	39.7g	0.5g	0.5g

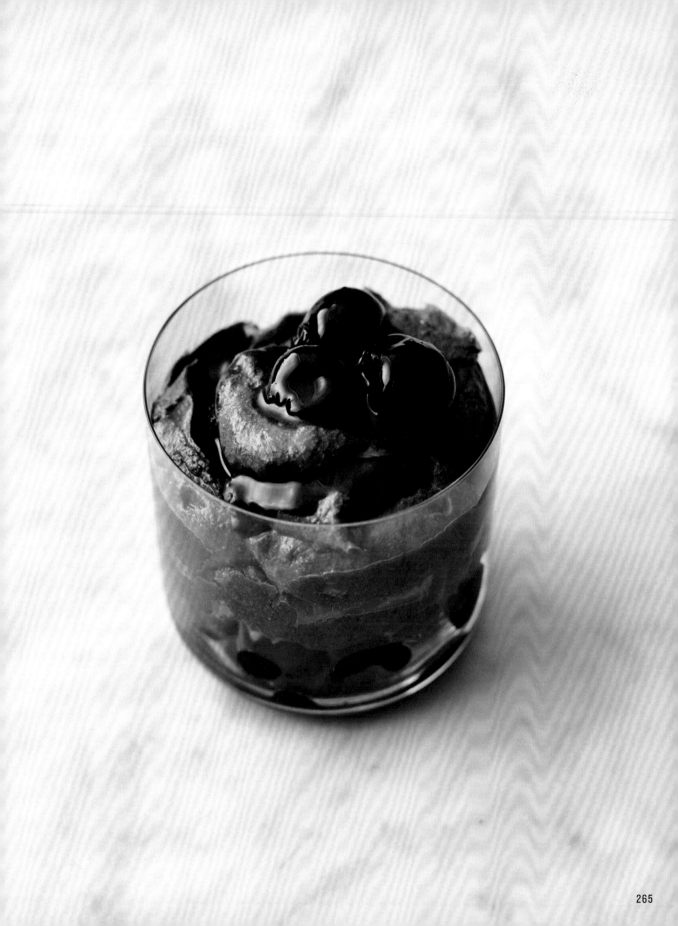

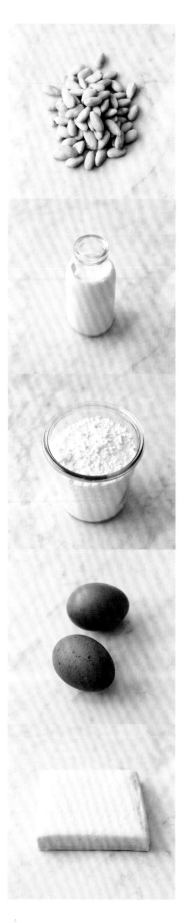

ALMOND PASTRY PUFF

SERVES 6   TOTAL 28 MINUTES

100g blanched almonds

1 tablespoon double cream, plus extra to serve

75g icing sugar, plus extra for dusting

2 large eggs

375g block of all-butter puff pastry (cold)

Preheat the oven to 220°C/425°F/gas 7. Line a baking tray with greaseproof paper. Blitz the almonds in a food processor until nice and fine. With the processor still running, add the cream, icing sugar, 1 egg and a pinch of sea salt until combined, stopping to scrape down the sides with a spatula, if needed.

Halve the pastry, shape into two rounds and, working quickly, dusting with icing sugar as you go to stop the pastry sticking, roll out between two sheets of greaseproof paper until they're just under ½cm thick. Place one round on the lined tray. Spread the almond paste on top, leaving a 2cm gap at the edges. Put the other round on top and gently push together. Quickly seal the edges with the back of a fork. Eggwash the top, then dust over an extra layer of sugar.

Gently push your finger into the middle of the pastry, then, with a sharp knife, very delicately make little lines from the centre to the outside. Bake on the bottom of the oven for 12 to 15 minutes, or until puffed up and golden, dusting with a little extra icing sugar before dishing up.

CALORIES	FAT	SAT FAT	PROTEIN	CARBS	SUGAR	SALT	FIBRE
443kcal	29.2g	12.7g	8.9g	36.7g	14.7g	0.7g	0.9g

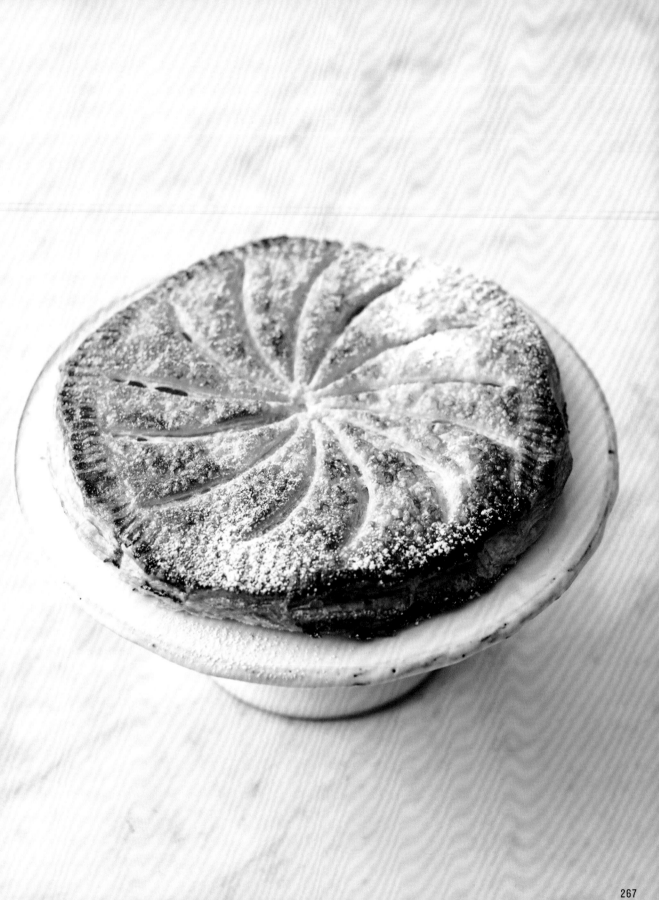

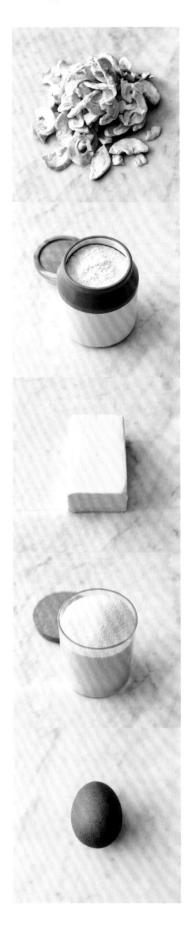

APPLE CRUMBLE COOKIES

MAKES 24 | TOTAL 24 MINUTES

100g dried apple

200g self-raising flour

100g unsalted butter (cold)

100g golden caster sugar

1 large egg

Preheat the oven to 200°C/400°F/gas 6. Line two trays with greaseproof paper and rub with olive oil. Whiz the apple in a food processor until finely chopped, then add the flour, cubed butter, sugar and a pinch of sea salt. Blitz to fine crumbs for 1 minute, then remove 3 tablespoons of the mix and set aside. Pulse in the egg until combined, stopping to scrape down the sides, if needed.

Divide into 24 pieces, roll into balls, then press down lightly into 4cm rounds, lining them up on the trays as you go. Sprinkle over the reserved mix, lightly pressing it into the cookies. Bake for 8 to 10 minutes, or until lightly golden. Leave to cool slightly, then transfer to a wire cooling rack. Yum!

CALORIES	FAT	SAT FAT	PROTEIN	CARBS	SUGAR	SALT	FIBRE
89kcal	3.8g	2.2g	1.1g	13.1g	6.9g	0.2g	0.7g

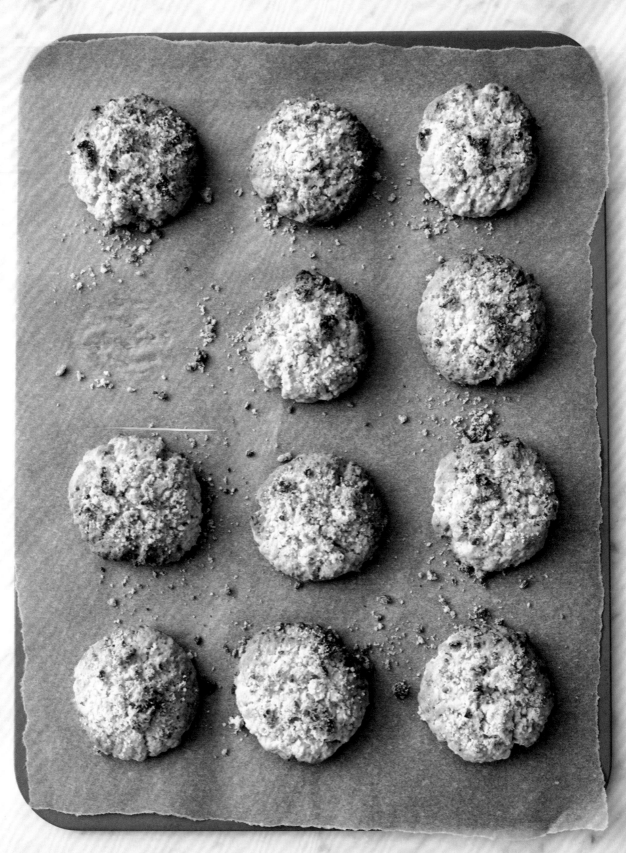

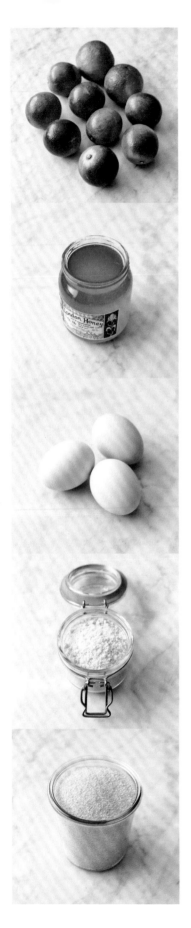

ORANGE POLENTA CAKE

SERVES 8-10 | FAST PREP 10 MINUTES | COOK + COOL 50 MINUTES

10 regular or blood oranges

250g runny honey

3 large eggs

200g ground almonds

100g fine polenta

Preheat the oven to 160°C/325°F/gas 3. Rub a 20cm springform cake tin with olive oil, then line the base with greaseproof paper and rub the paper with oil, too. Squeeze the juice of 3 oranges (roughly 100ml) into a pan, add 100g of honey and simmer until thickened and reduced, then remove from the heat.

Meanwhile, in a free-standing mixer on a high speed, whisk 200ml of olive oil with the remaining 150g of honey for 2 minutes to combine. Beat in the eggs for 2 minutes, while you finely grate and add the zest of 3 oranges. Stop the mixer, then fold in the ground almonds, polenta, and the juice of 1 or 2 oranges (roughly 50ml). Pour into the prepared tin and bake for 40 to 50 minutes, or until golden and cooked through. Leave to cool for 10 minutes in the tin, loosening with a palette knife before releasing – be gentle with it.

To serve, quickly peel and slice the remaining oranges and dish up alongside the cake, drizzling the pretty syrup over everything before tucking in.

CALORIES	FAT	SAT FAT	PROTEIN	CARBS	SUGAR	SALT	FIBRE
490kcal	33.4g	4.4g	8.4g	41.2g	32.8g	0.1g	2g

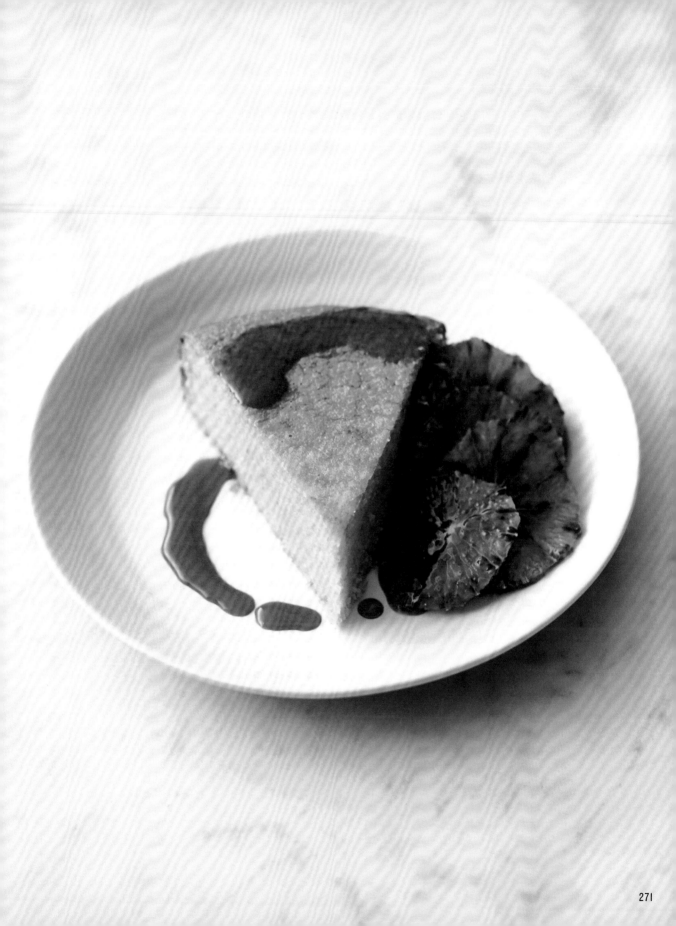

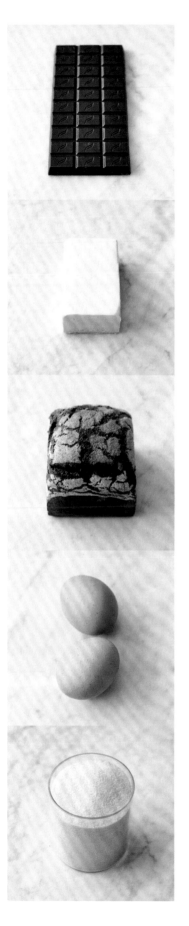

CHOCOLATE RYE COOKIES

MAKES 24 | TOTAL 28 MINUTES

100g dark chocolate (70%)

100g unsalted butter

100g rye bread

2 large eggs

50g golden caster sugar

Preheat the oven to 200°C/400°F/gas 6. Line two trays with greaseproof paper and rub with olive oil. Melt the chocolate in a heatproof bowl over a pan of gently simmering water, then remove and stir in the butter so it melts. Tear the bread into a food processor and blitz into fine crumbs, then add the eggs and sugar, and blitz again well. With the processor still running, pour in the chocolate mixture and let it blitz until combined.

Spoon the cookie mix into a large sandwich bag, snip off the corner and pipe 3–4cm blobs to make 24 cookies on the lined trays. Bake for 8 to 10 minutes, or until spread and set. Sprinkle with sea salt, leave to cool a little, and tuck in.

CALORIES	FAT	SAT FAT	PROTEIN	CARBS	SUGAR	SALT	FIBRE
76kcal	5.2g	3g	1.2g	6.8g	4.9g	0.2g	0.2g

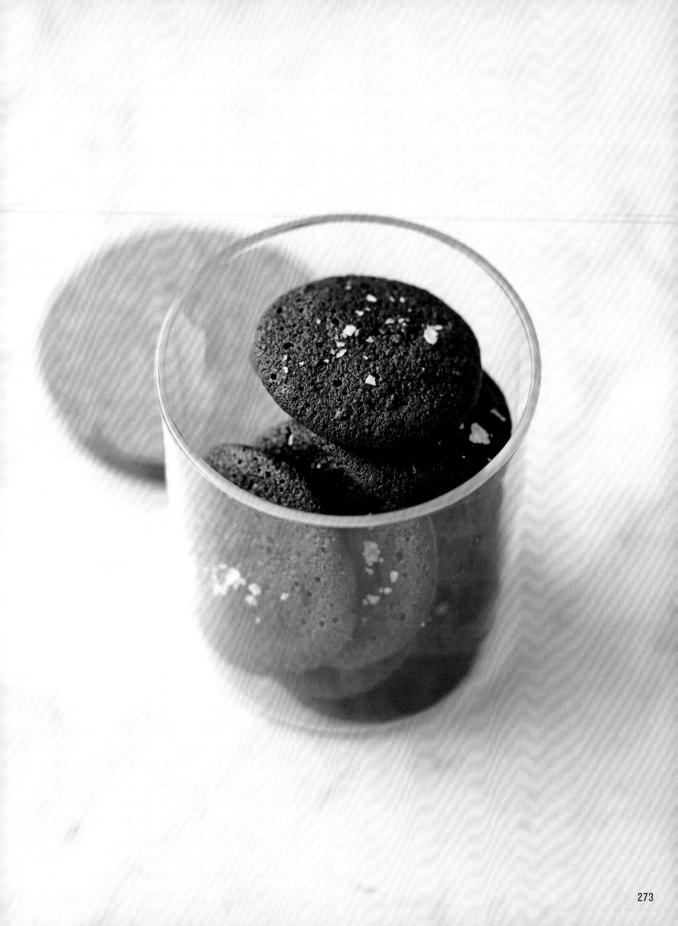

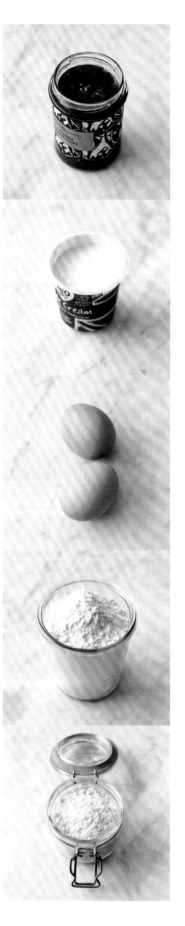

SPEEDY STEAMED PUDDING POTS

SERVES 6   TOTAL 17 MINUTES

375g chunky marmalade

150ml single cream, plus extra to serve

2 large eggs

100g self-raising flour

150g ground almonds

Grease six heatproof teacups with a little olive oil. In a large bowl, whisk 100ml of olive oil and 2 tablespoons of marmalade with the cream and eggs. Add the flour, almonds and a pinch of sea salt, and whisk again to combine. Place the remaining marmalade in a small pan with a splash of water and simmer on a medium-high heat until thick and syrupy, then remove.

Divide the pudding mixture between the teacups, then microwave in pairs for 2½ to 3 minutes on high, or until puffed up. Turn out, drizzle with the marmalade syrup, and serve with a little extra cream, if you like.

CALORIES	FAT	SAT FAT	PROTEIN	CARBS	SUGAR	SALT	FIBRE
596kcal	37.6g	7.1g	10g	58.3g	45.3g	0.3g	0.9g

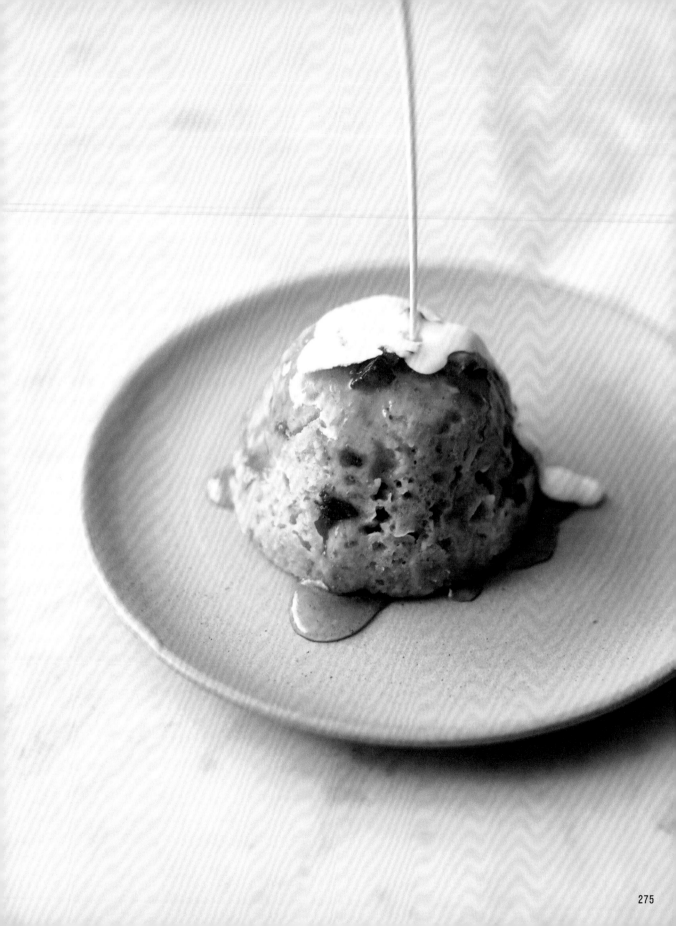

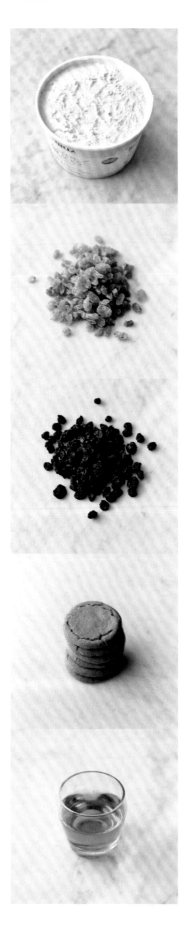

FLAMING RUM 'N' RAISIN

SERVES 4   TOTAL JUST 10 MINUTES

4 large scoops of vanilla ice cream

60g golden sultanas

60g raisins

6 ginger nut biscuits

100ml dark spiced rum

Get your ice cream out of the freezer. Put the sultanas, raisins and a splash of water into a pan on a medium heat, so they plump up for a few minutes as the water evaporates. Meanwhile, smash up the biscuits in a pestle and mortar and divide between four bowls, adding a nice round ball of ice cream to each.

When the water's gone, pour the rum over the sultanas and raisins and carefully set fire to it with a match, if you like (stand back!). Once the flames begin to subside, spoon the mixture over your ice cream balls. Heaven.

CALORIES	FAT	SAT FAT	PROTEIN	CARBS	SUGAR	SALT	FIBRE
289kcal	6.6g	3.7g	3g	43.1g	36.5g	0.3g	0.4g

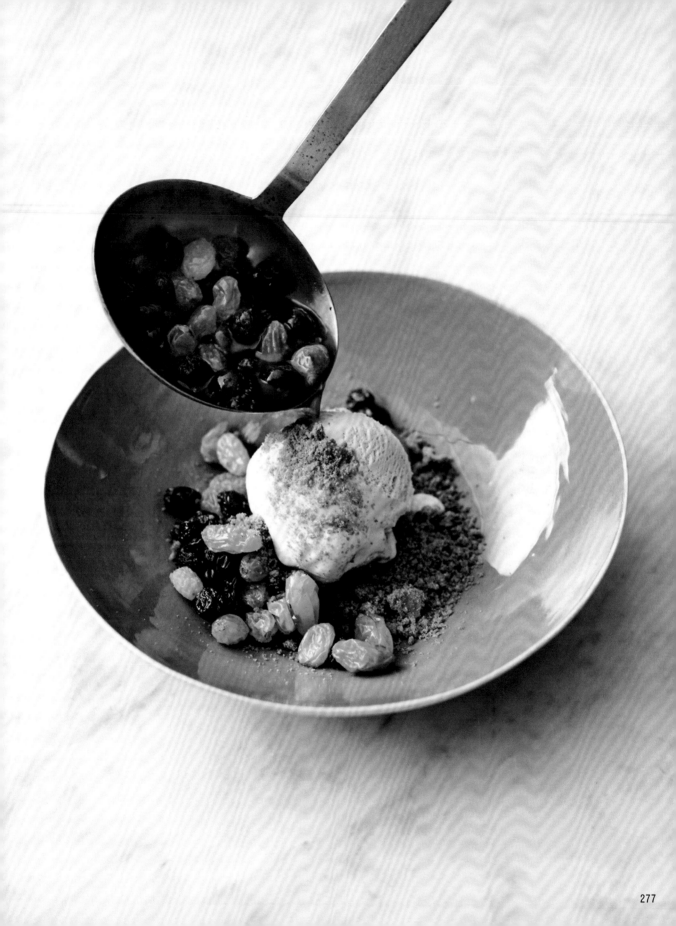

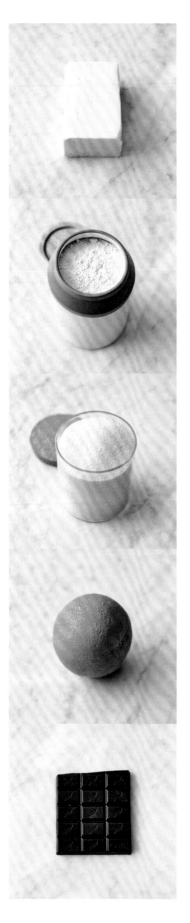

CHOCOLATE ORANGE SHORTBREAD

MAKES 12   TOTAL 30 MINUTES

150g unsalted butter (at room temperature)

200g plain flour

50g golden caster sugar, plus extra to sprinkle

1 orange

50g dark chocolate (70%)

Preheat the oven to 190°C/375°F/gas 5. Grease a 20cm square baking tin and line with greaseproof paper. In a bowl, mix together the butter, flour, sugar and the finely grated zest of half the orange by rubbing the mixture between your thumbs and fingertips. Squash and pat into dough – don't knead it – then push into the lined tin in a 1cm-thick layer. Prick all over with a fork, then bake for 20 minutes, or until lightly golden. Remove, sprinkle over a little extra sugar while it's still warm, then leave to cool.

Meanwhile, melt the chocolate in a heatproof bowl over a pan of gently simmering water, then remove. Cut the shortbread into 12 finger portions, then transfer to a wire cooling rack. Drizzle with the chocolate, then finely grate over the remaining orange zest. Cut up the orange, and serve on the side!

CALORIES	FAT	SAT FAT	PROTEIN	CARBS	SUGAR	SALT	FIBRE
188kcal	11.6g	7.3g	1.9g	20g	7.3g	0g	0.6g

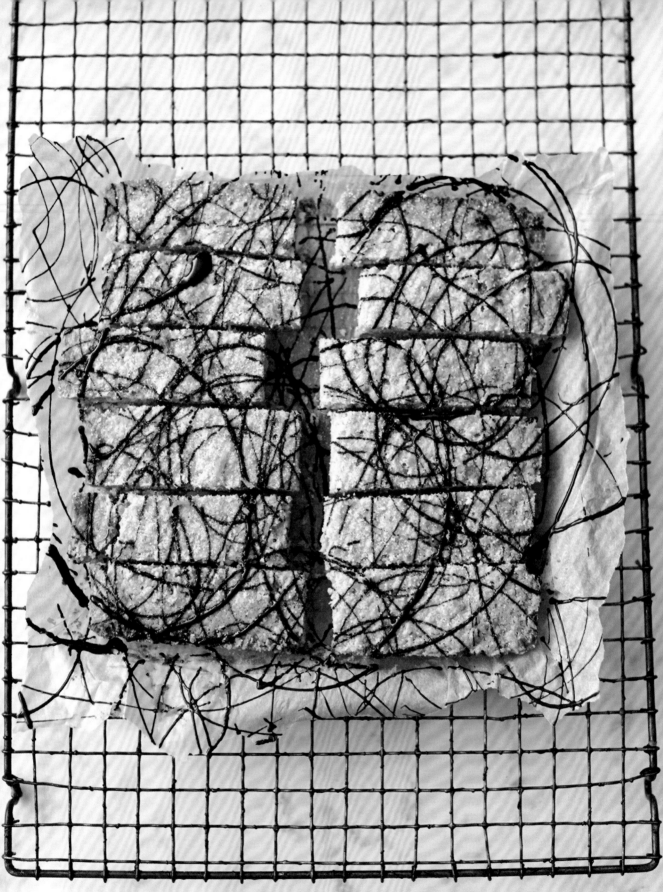

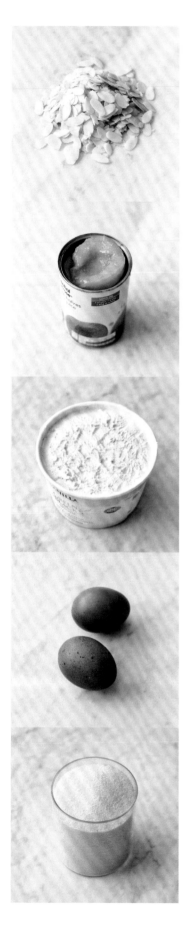

PEACH & ALMOND ALASKA

SERVES 4   TOTAL 26 MINUTES

80g flaked almonds

1 x 410g tin of peach halves in juice

4 large scoops of vanilla ice cream

2 large eggs

100g golden caster sugar

Preheat the grill to high. Toast the almonds on a tray as it heats up, keeping a close eye on them and removing as soon as lightly golden. Slice up the peaches and divide between four ovenproof bowls, along with their juice. Sit a nice round scoop of ice cream on top of each, and place in the freezer.

Separate the eggs. Put the whites into the bowl of a free-standing mixer (save the yolks for another recipe), add a pinch of sea salt and whisk until the mixture forms stiff peaks (you could use an electric hand whisk). With the mixer still running, gradually add the sugar until combined. Spoon into a piping bag (I like a star-shaped nozzle) or a large sandwich bag that you can snip the corner off.

Remove the bowls from the freezer and scatter over the toasted almonds. Pipe the meringue over the ice cream as delicately or roughly as you like. Now – I work two at a time to retain maximum control – pop the bowls under the grill for just 2 minutes, or until golden. Remove carefully and serve right away.

CALORIES	FAT	SAT FAT	PROTEIN	CARBS	SUGAR	SALT	FIBRE
386kcal	18.4g	4.3g	10g	48.6g	48g	0.7g	0.1g

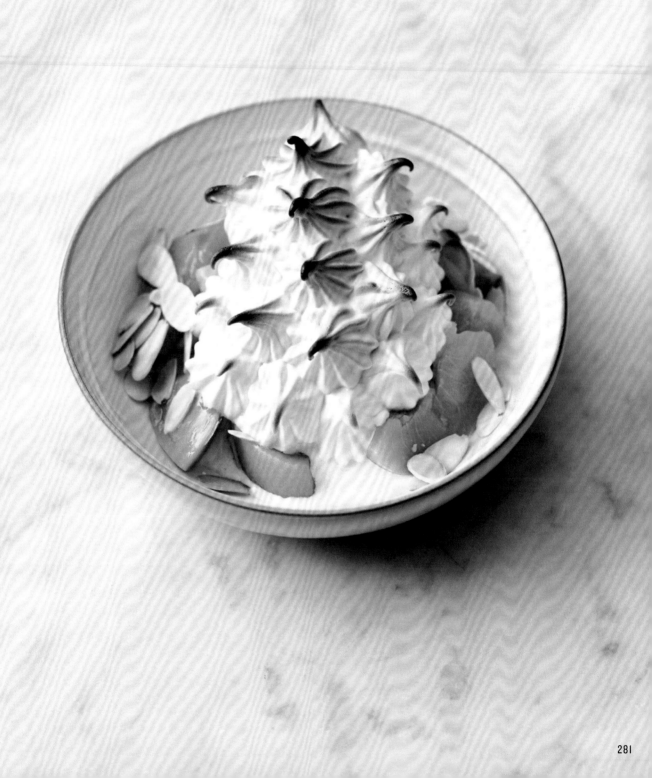

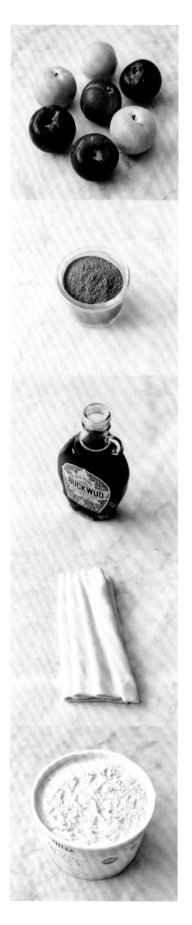

PLUM TARTE TATIN

SERVES 6 | TOTAL 24 MINUTES

600g ripe mixed-colour plums

1 teaspoon ground cinnamon

120ml maple syrup

320g sheet of all-butter puff pastry (cold)

6 large scoops of vanilla ice cream

Preheat the oven to 220°C/425°F/gas 7. Place a 26cm non-stick ovenproof frying pan on a medium heat. Halve and destone the plums, add to the pan with 30ml of water, and cook for 1 minute. From a height, sprinkle over half the cinnamon, then evenly pour over the maple syrup. Place the pastry over the plums, using a wooden spoon to push it into the edges of the pan, and trimming off any excess to patch up little gaps, if needed.

Bake at the bottom of the oven for 16 minutes, or until golden and puffed up. Making sure you use oven gloves to protect your hands, confidently and very carefully turn the tarte out on to a plate bigger than the pan. Dish up with nice round scoops of ice cream, sprinkle over the remaining cinnamon from a height and drizzle lightly with extra virgin olive oil before serving.

CALORIES	FAT	SAT FAT	PROTEIN	CARBS	SUGAR	SALT	FIBRE
392kcal	18.7g	11.8g	4.8g	52.3g	32.8g	0.3g	1.2g

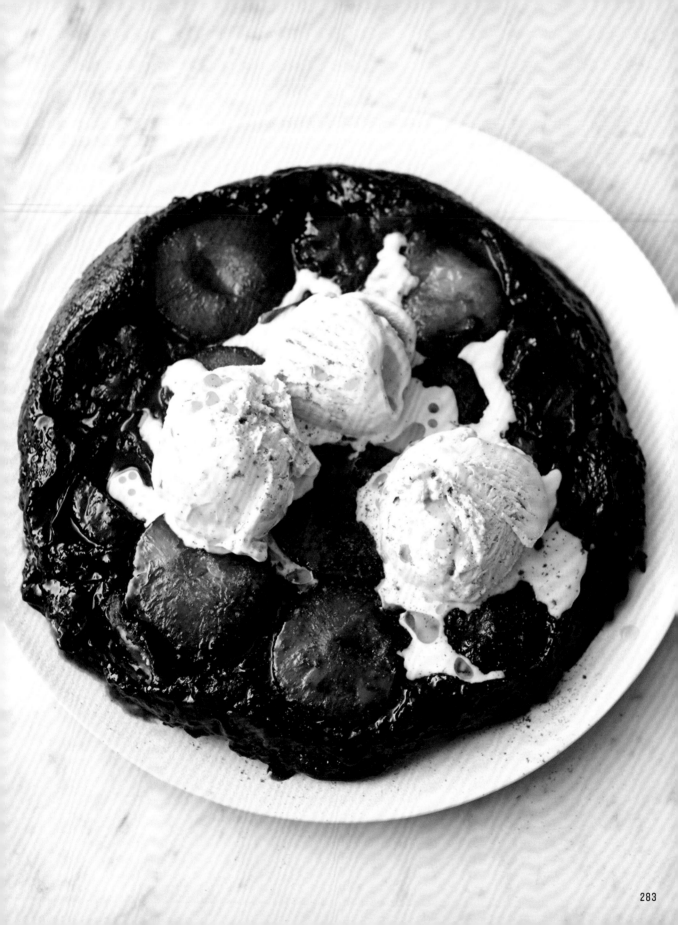

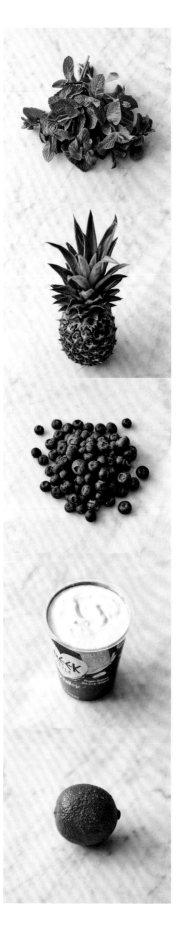

PINEAPPLE CARPACCIO

SERVES 4   TOTAL JUST 10 MINUTES

1 bunch of fresh mint (30g)

1 ripe pineapple

100g blueberries

4 tablespoons Greek-style coconut yoghurt

1 lime

Pick the mint leaves into a pestle and mortar, reserving a small handful of leaves to one side. Pound the rest into a paste, then muddle in 1 to 2 tablespoons of extra virgin olive oil to make a mint oil. Top and tail the pineapple, then slice off the skin. Quarter lengthways, remove the core, then finely slice lengthways. Arrange on a large platter or divide between your plates. Take the time to halve the blueberries, then sprinkle over the top.

Ripple some mint oil through the yoghurt (saving the rest for another recipe), then spoon over the fruit. Finely grate over the lime zest from a height and squeeze over the juice. Finely slice and sprinkle over the reserved mint leaves, then drizzle with a tiny bit of extra virgin olive oil (yes, you heard it – delicious).

CALORIES	FAT	SAT FAT	PROTEIN	CARBS	SUGAR	SALT	FIBRE
122kcal	5.6g	2.5g	1.3g	17.5g	15.4g	0g	0.4g

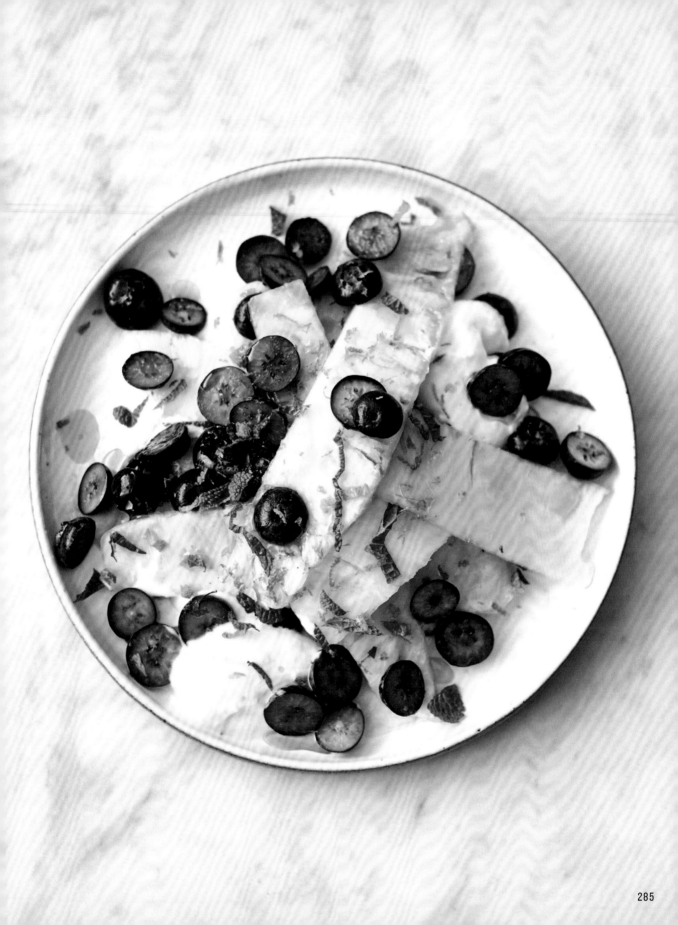

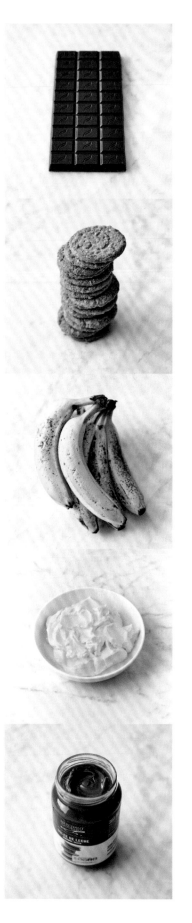

FROZEN BANOFFEE CHEESECAKE

SERVES 10   TOTAL PREP 18 MINUTES   FREEZE OVERNIGHT

150g dark chocolate (70%)

300g packet of Hobnobs

8 overripe bananas

500g light cream cheese

½ x 450g jar of dulce de leche

Rub the base of a 20cm springform cake tin with olive oil and line with greaseproof paper, then rub the paper with oil, too. Melt 50g of chocolate in a heatproof bowl over a pan of gently simmering water, then remove. Snap the Hobnobs into a food processor and blitz with 2 tablespoons of extra virgin olive oil until well combined. Drizzle in the melted chocolate, then pulse again. Pat into the cake tin in a 1cm-thick layer.

Peel the bananas, tear into the food processor, add the cream cheese and dulce de leche, blitz well until nice and smooth, then pour over the biscuit base. Freeze overnight or until needed, transferring to the fridge for 2 hours before serving, or until it's the slicing consistency you like.

Loosen the edges of the cheesecake with a palette knife, then release from the tin. Shave or grate over the remaining chocolate, and serve. Delicious.

CALORIES	FAT	SAT FAT	PROTEIN	CARBS	SUGAR	SALT	FIBRE
482kcal	22g	8.1g	9.6g	63.5g	48.7g	0.8g	3.1g

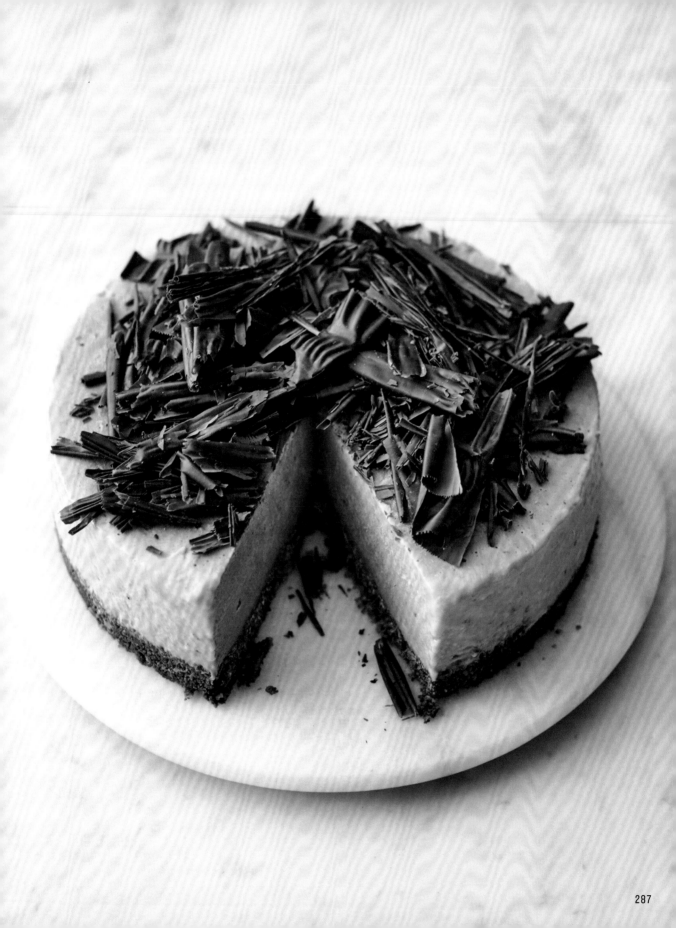

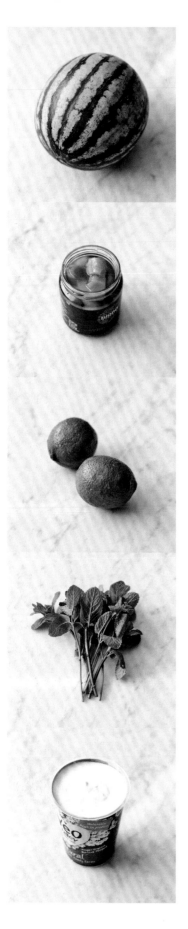

WATERMELON GRANITA

SERVES 8 | TOTAL PREP 14 MINUTES | FREEZE 8 HOURS

1 small watermelon (1.8kg)

60g stem ginger in syrup

2 limes

½ a bunch of fresh mint (15g)

8 tablespoons natural yoghurt

Cut off the watermelon rind, then chop the flesh into chunks, picking out any seeds. Roughly chop the ginger and place in a large sealable freezer bag with the watermelon chunks. Finely grate in the lime zest, squeeze in all the juice, then freeze flat for at least 8 hours, or until super-hard.

When ready to serve, pick and reserve the baby mint leaves, then pick the rest into a food processor. Tip in the frozen watermelon mixture and blitz to a pink snow (in batches, if you need to). Serve 2 heaped tablespoons of granita per person, with 1 tablespoon of yoghurt, a drizzle of ginger syrup from the jar and a few baby mint leaves. It's nice to use chilled plates, bowls or glasses here.

CALORIES	FAT	SAT FAT	PROTEIN	CARBS	SUGAR	SALT	FIBRE
109kcal	1.6g	0.8g	2.2g	22.7g	22.4g	0.1g	0g

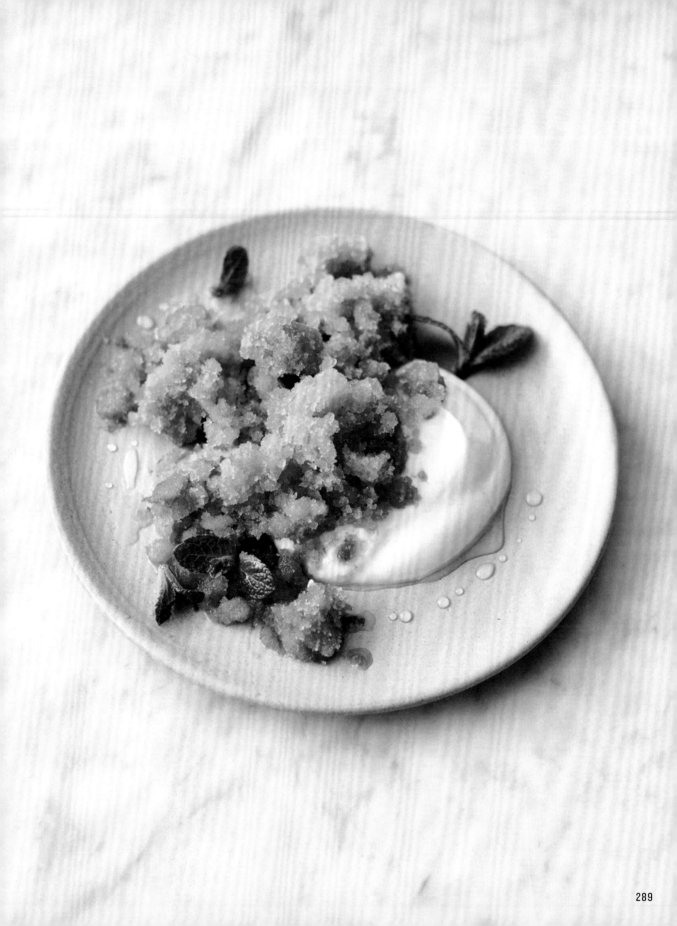

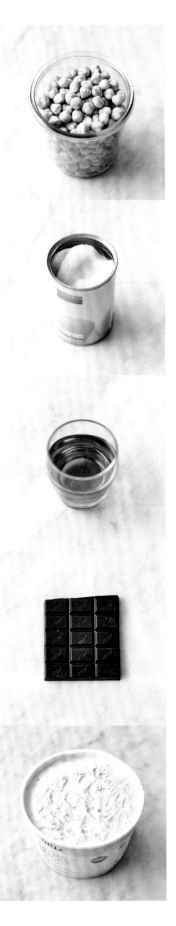

BOOZY PEARS & CHOCOLATE

SERVES 4   TOTAL JUST 15 MINUTES

40g blanched hazelnuts

1 x 410g tin of pear halves in juice

50ml Armagnac

50g dark chocolate (70%)

4 large scoops of vanilla ice cream

Toast the hazelnuts in a large non-stick frying pan on a high heat for 2 minutes, until lightly golden, tossing regularly, then tip into a pestle and mortar, returning the pan to the heat. Pour in the pears (juice and all), let them get hot, then add the Armagnac. Stand back and carefully set light to the liquor with a match. Let it flame, then leave to bubble and reduce to a lovely syrup. Meanwhile, crush the hazelnuts and divide between four plates, making a pile on each one.

Spoon the pears on to the plates, cup side up. Remove the syrup from the heat, then snap most of the chocolate into the pan. While it melts, top each hazelnut pile with a nice round scoop of ice cream, and shave over the last bit of chocolate. Mix up the chocolate syrup, drizzle into the pear cups, and serve.

CALORIES	FAT	SAT FAT	PROTEIN	CARBS	SUGAR	SALT	FIBRE
275kcal	14g	5.2g	3.9g	28.3g	27.9g	0.1g	0.8g

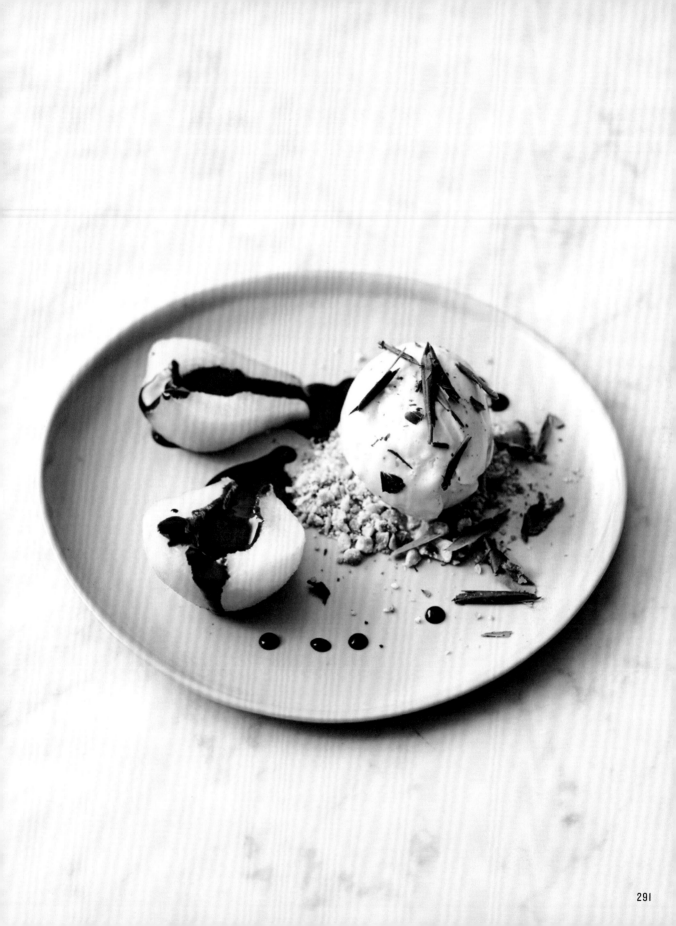

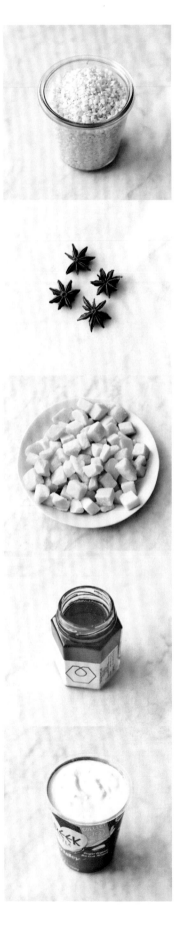

MANGO RICE PUDDING

SERVES 4   TOTAL 28 MINUTES

150g pudding rice

4 star anise

350g frozen mango chunks

4 tablespoons runny honey

4 tablespoons Greek-style coconut yoghurt

Place the rice, star anise, frozen mango, 3 tablespoons of honey and a tiny pinch of sea salt in a pan on a medium heat. Cover with 700ml of water and simmer for 25 minutes, or until thick and creamy, stirring occasionally.

Stir through the yoghurt so it's nice and creamy, then divide between your bowls. Drizzle over the remaining honey, and enjoy. Super-easy!

CALORIES	FAT	SAT FAT	PROTEIN	CARBS	SUGAR	SALT	FIBRE
276kcal	3g	2.2g	3.5g	63.2g	29.4g	0.2g	0.6g

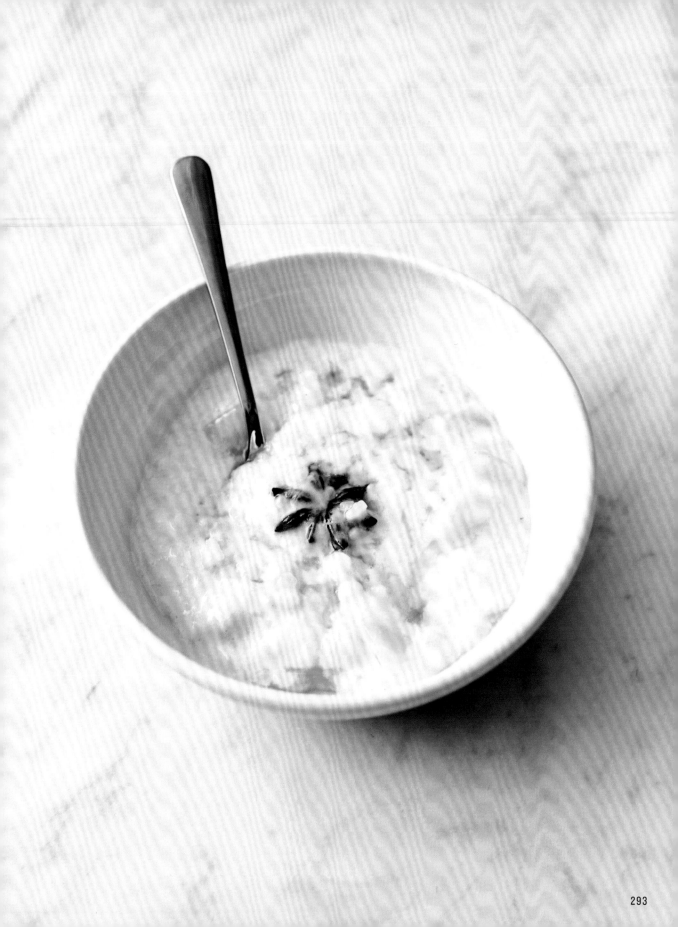

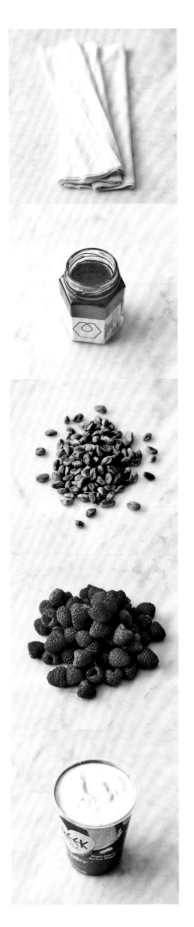

HONEY BERRY FILO SMASH

SERVES 4   TOTAL JUST 14 MINUTES

3 sheets of filo pastry

6 heaped teaspoons runny honey

40g shelled pistachios

200g raspberries

400g Greek-style coconut yoghurt

Preheat the oven to 180°C/350°F/gas 4. Lay 1 sheet of filo on an oiled baking tray, drizzle with 1 heaped teaspoon of honey from a height, then repeat. Lay the final sheet of filo over the top and drizzle with a little olive oil. Scatter over the pistachios, then bake for 10 minutes, or until everything is golden. Meanwhile, crush half the raspberries with a fork and ripple them through the yoghurt, then divide between your plates.

Shake the pistachios on to a board, then lightly crush. Snap off pieces of crispy filo and arrange nicely on top of the yoghurt. Scatter over the pistachios and remaining raspberries, then drizzle over the remaining honey from a height.

CALORIES	FAT	SAT FAT	PROTEIN	CARBS	SUGAR	SALT	FIBRE
359kcal	18g	11.2g	6.6g	45g	18.4g	0.4g	2g

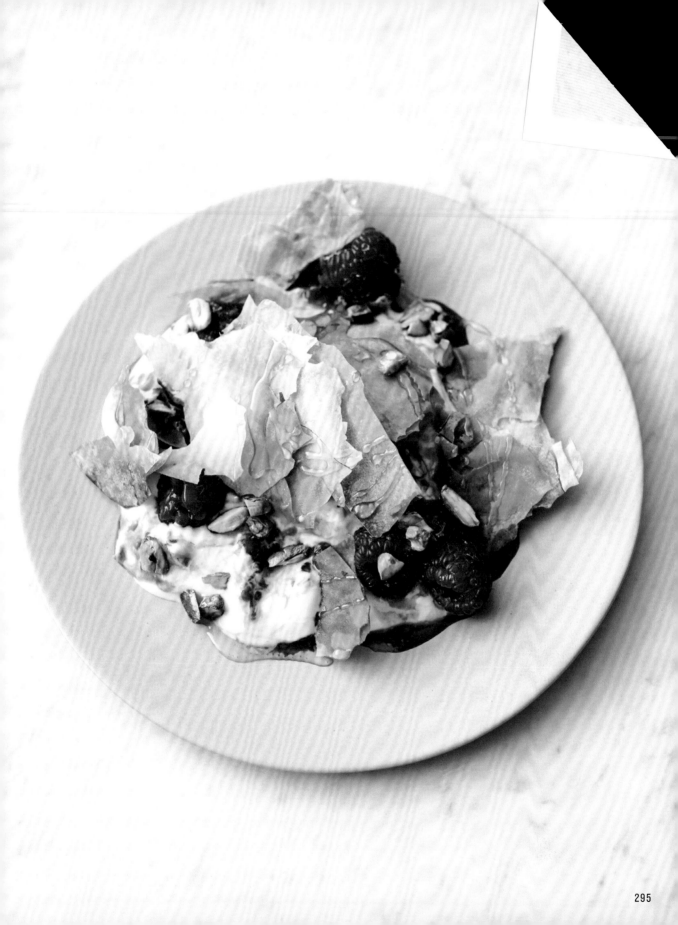

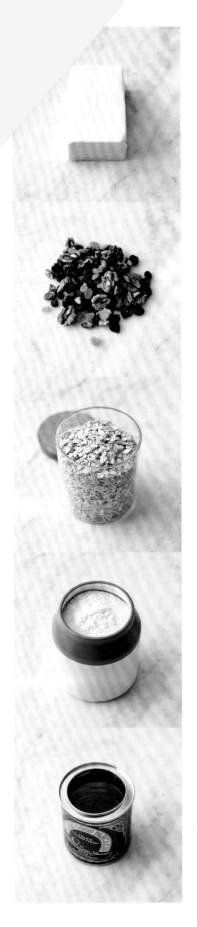

BUDDY'S FLAPJACK BISCUITS

MAKES 16   TOTAL 29 MINUTES

100g unsalted butter (at room temperature)

100g mixed dried fruit & nuts

100g porridge oats

100g self-raising flour

100g golden syrup

Preheat the oven to 180°C/350°F/gas 4. Line a deep 20cm square baking tin with greaseproof paper and rub with olive oil. Pulse the butter, dried fruit and nuts, oats and flour in a food processor until the mix comes together and away from the sides, then pulse in the syrup until fully combined.

Transfer to the lined tin, flattening to the edges. Bake for 15 to 20 minutes, or until golden. Remove from the oven, slice into 16 squares ready to cut, and leave to cool in the tin for 5 minutes. Use the paper to lift out on to a wire rack, and leave to cool completely. Simple, easy, delicious – spread the word!

CALORIES	FAT	SAT FAT	PROTEIN	CARBS	SUGAR	SALT	FIBRE
140kcal	7.9g	3.8g	2.1g	16.1g	6.9g	0.1g	1g

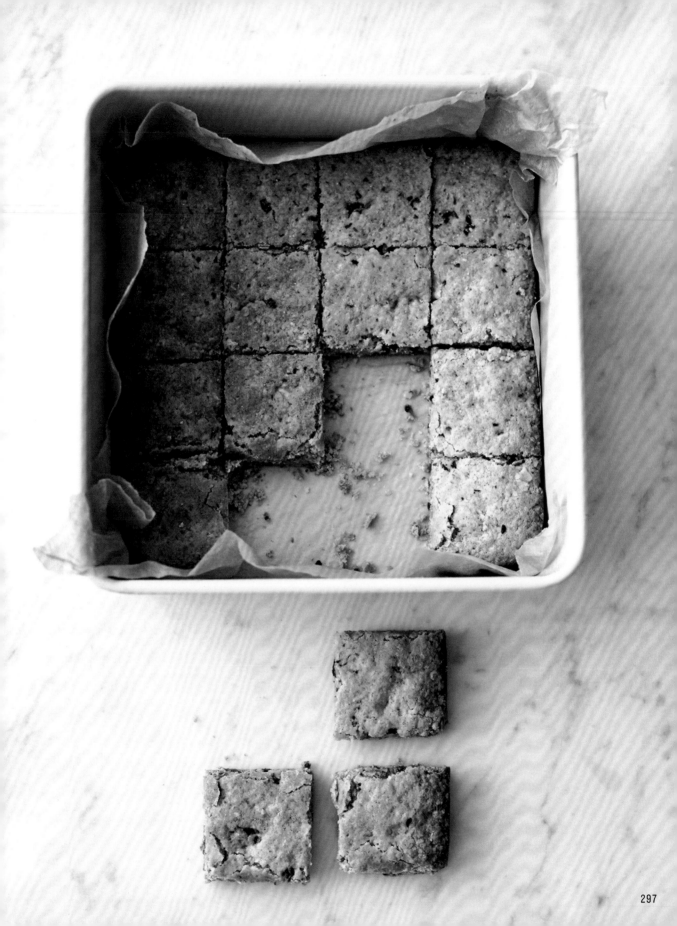

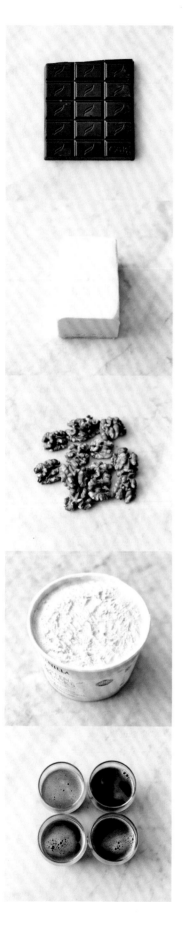

WALNUT-WHIP AFFOGATO

SERVES 4   TOTAL JUST 9 MINUTES

50g dark chocolate (70%)

20g unsalted butter

50g shelled unsalted walnut halves

4 large scoops of vanilla ice cream

4 long shots of espresso

Melt the chocolate and butter with a pinch of sea salt in a heatproof bowl over a pan of gently simmering water, then remove. Reserving 4 perfect walnut halves for decoration, slice or crumble up the rest.

Roll your ice cream into nice round scoops and divide between four teacups. Scatter over the sliced or crumbled walnuts, pour a shot of hot espresso into each cup, stick a walnut proudly on top, then drizzle over the melted chocolate.

CALORIES	FAT	SAT FAT	PROTEIN	CARBS	SUGAR	SALT	FIBRE
272kcal	20.3g	8.2g	4.2g	19.5g	19.3g	0.6g	4.2g

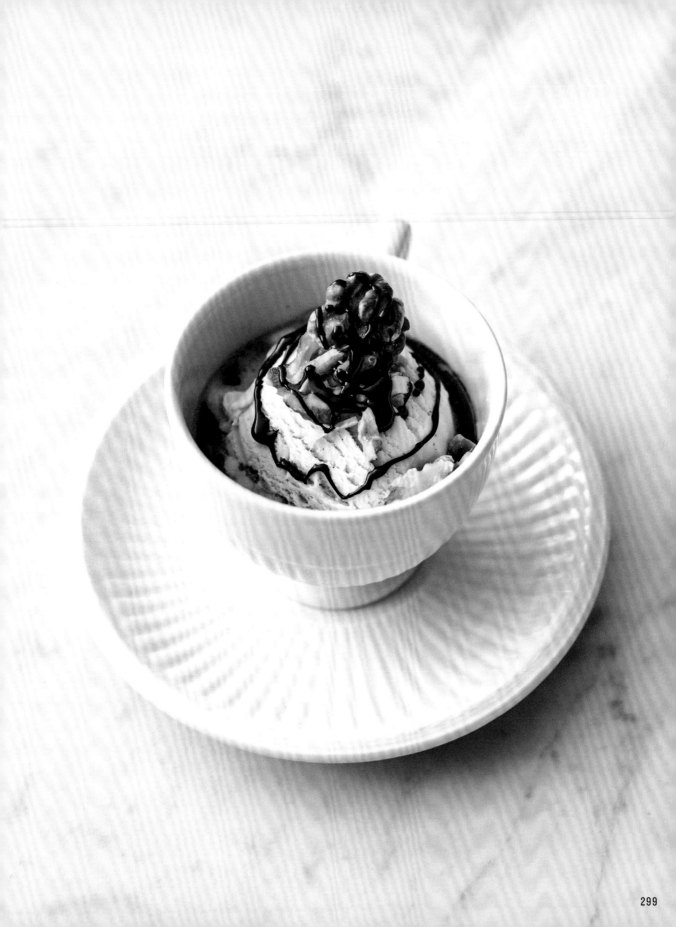

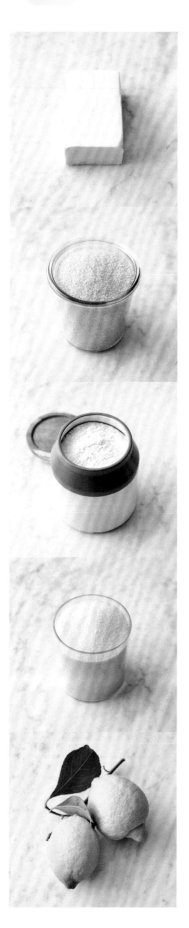

ST CLEMENT'S POLENTA BISCUITS

MAKES 24   TOTAL 28 MINUTES

100g unsalted butter (cold)

50g fine polenta

150g self-raising flour

100g golden caster sugar, plus extra to sprinkle

2 lemons (or oranges)

Preheat the oven to 180°C/350°F/gas 4. Line two trays with greaseproof paper and rub with olive oil. Cube the butter and place in a food processor with the polenta, flour and sugar. Finely grate in the zest of 1 lemon (or orange), then pulse to combine. Squeeze in the juice of half a lemon (or orange), and pulse again to bring the mixture together into a ball of dough.

Divide into 24 pieces, roll into balls and place on the trays, leaving a 5cm gap between them. With your thumb, create a 1cm-deep dent in the centre of each ball. Finely grate the remaining lemon (or orange) zest and scatter into the dents, followed by a little sprinkle of caster sugar. Bake for 10 minutes, or until lightly golden. Transfer to a wire rack to cool, then tuck in.

CALORIES	FAT	SAT FAT	PROTEIN	CARBS	SUGAR	SALT	FIBRE
70kcal	3.6g	2.2g	0.7g	9.4g	4.4g	0.1g	0.2g

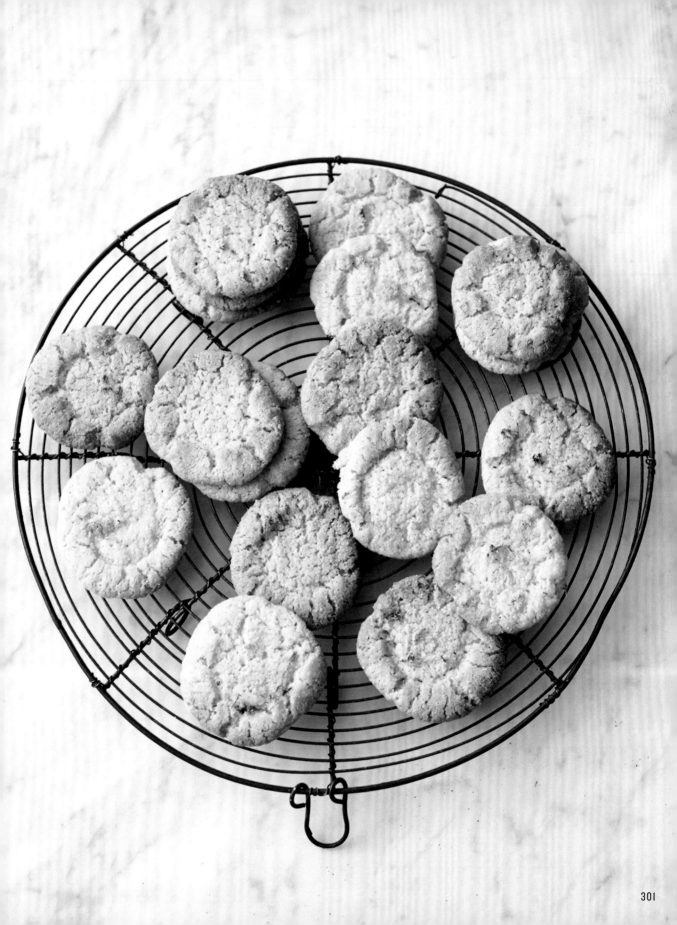

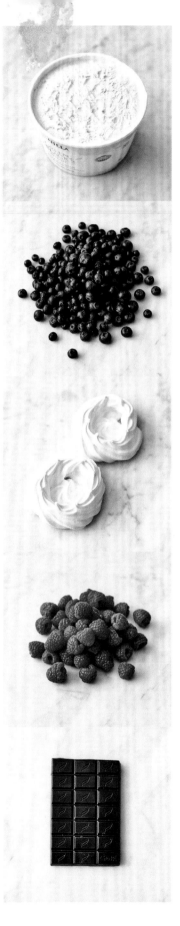

BERRY MERINGUE RIPPLE

SERVES 2 | TOTAL JUST 8 MINUTES

2 large scoops of vanilla ice cream

200g blueberries

2 shop-bought meringues

100g raspberries

dark chocolate (70%), to serve

Get your ice cream out of the freezer. Put the blueberries into a non-stick frying pan with a splash of water and place on a high heat for 2 minutes, or until they all start to burst and get jammy, then remove from the heat.

Layering up as you like, crumble the meringues between glasses or bowls, halve and add the raspberries and a nice round scoop of ice cream to each, then spoon over the jammy blueberries and their juices. Shave or grate over a little chocolate and tuck in, rippling it all together in a wonderful collision of flavours.

CALORIES	FAT	SAT FAT	PROTEIN	CARBS	SUGAR	SALT	FIBRE
250kcal	7.2g	4.3g	4.7g	44.lg	44g	0.lg	l.6g

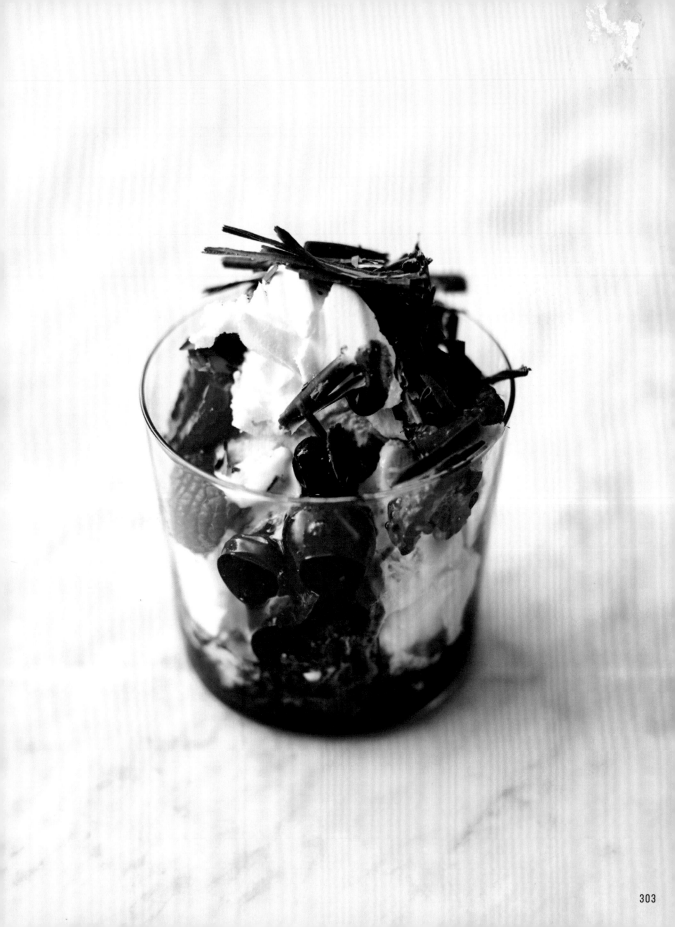

Our job is to make sure that Jamie can be super-creative, while also ensuring that all his recipes meet the guidelines we set. With the exception of the sweet treats chapter, 70% of the recipes in this book fit into our healthy guidelines, but they're not all complete meals, so you'll need to balance out your mealtimes with what's lacking. So that you can make informed choices, we've published the nutritional content for each recipe on the recipe page itself, giving you an easy access point to understand what you're eating. Remember – a good, balanced diet and regular exercise are the keys to a healthier lifestyle. For more info about our guidelines and how we analyse recipes, please visit **jamieoliver.com/nutrition**.

Laura Matthews – Head of Nutrition, RNutr (food)

THE BALANCED PLATE

Balance is key when it comes to eating well. Balance your plate right and keep your portion control in check, and you can be confident that you're giving yourself a great start on the path to good health.

You don't have to be spot-on every day – just try to get your balance right across the week. If you eat meat and fish, as a general guide for main meals you want at least two portions of fish a week, one of which should be oily. Split the rest of the week's main meals between brilliant plant-based meals, some poultry and a little red meat. An all-vegetarian diet can be perfectly healthy, too.

HOW TO BALANCE YOUR PLATE

The easiest way is to follow UK government guidelines from Public Health England. Check out the exact percentages they recommend below, and how to think about the proportion of food on your plate.

THE FIVE FOOD GROUPS (UK)	PROPORTION OF YOUR PLATE
Vegetables and fruit	Just over one-third (40%)
Starchy carbohydrates (bread, rice, potatoes, pasta)	Just over one-third (38%)
Protein (meat, fish, eggs, beans, other non-dairy sources)	Around one-eighth (12%)
Dairy foods, milk & dairy alternatives	Around one-eighth (8%)
Unsaturated fats (such as oils)	Use in small amounts (1%)

AND DON'T FORGET TO DRINK PLENTY OF WATER, TOO

This nutritional bounty, laden with vitamins and minerals, should sit right at the heart of your diet. Wonderful veg and fruit come in all kinds of shapes, sizes, colours, flavours and textures. Eat the rainbow, mixing up your choices as much as you can and embracing the seasons so you're getting produce at its best and its most nutritious. As an absolute minimum, aim for five 80g portions of fresh, frozen or tinned veg and fruit every day of the week, enjoying more, wherever possible. You can also count one 30g portion of dried fruit, one 80g portion of beans or pulses, and one 150ml serving of unsweetened veg or fruit juice per day.

Carbs make us feel happy and satisfied, and, crucially, provide us with a large proportion of the energy needed to make our bodies move, and to ensure our organs have the fuel they need to function. When you can, choose fibre-rich wholegrain and wholewheat varieties, which take longer to break down, are slow-releasing and thus provide a more sustained level of energy, keeping you feeling fuller for longer. The average adult can have around 260g of carbohydrates a day, with up to 90g coming from total sugars. Fibre is also classed as a carbohydrate, and we should be aiming for about 30g of fibre each day.

This is an integral part of our diet, but one that does need to be controlled. Think of protein as the building blocks of our bodies – it's used for everything that's important to how we grow and repair. Generally, the optimal amount for women aged 19–50 is 45g per day, with 55g for men that are in the same age bracket.

This little slice of the balanced plate offers an amazing array of nutrients when eaten in the right amounts. Favour milk, yoghurt and small amounts of cheese in this category, and with milk and yoghurt, the lower-fat varieties (with no added sugar) are equally brilliant and worth embracing.

While we only need small amounts, we do require good fats. Choose unsaturated sources where you can, such as olive and liquid vegetable oils, nuts, seeds, avocado and omega-3-rich oily fish. Generally speaking, it's recommended that the average woman has no more than 70g of fat per day, with less than 20g of that from saturated fat, and the average man no more than 90g, with less than 30g from saturates.

This one is simple – to be the very best you can be, stay hydrated. Water is essential to life! In general, males aged 14 and over need at least 2.5 litres per day and females in the same age bracket need at least 2 litres per day.

Generally speaking, the average woman needs 2,000 calories a day, while the average man can have 2,500. These figures are a guide, and what we eat needs to be considered in relation to factors like age, build, lifestyle and activity levels. The good news is that all food and drinks can be eaten and drunk in moderation as part of a healthy, balanced diet, so we don't have to give up anything we really enjoy, unless advised to do so by a doctor or dietitian.

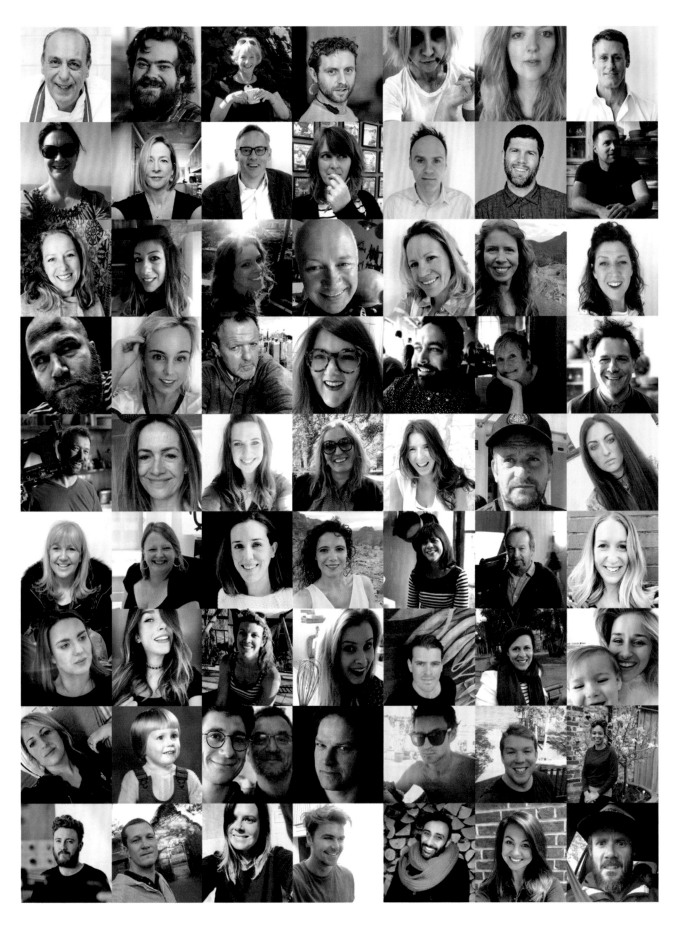

THANK YOU

I'm super-proud of this book, and particularly the way my brilliant teams and the wonderful people we work with externally jumped into action to make the *5-Ingredients* concept come to life, fast. You can see some of this amazing talent on the opposite page, and these lovely happy faces are just the tip of the iceberg. So, here goes . . .

Massive thanks to my supremely talented food team. To mother hen Ginny Rolfe, Abi 'Scottish' Fawcett, Christina 'Boochie' Mackenzie, Maddie Rix, Elspeth Allison, Jodene Jordan, Rachel Young, Jonny Lake, and to Simon Parkinson, Bella Williams and Becca Sulocki. To one-of-a-kind Mr Pete Begg, to Bobby Sebire, Sarah 'Tiddles' Tildesley, my Greek sister Georgina Hayden, Joanne Lewis, Athina Andrelos, Bianca Koffman, Barnaby Purdy, Ella Miller, Helen Martin and Daniel Nowland. To my talented nutritionists Laura Matthews and Rozzie Batchelar, thank you. To my epic girls on words, my editor Rebecca 'Rubs' Verity, Beth Stroud, Frances Stewart and the rest of the editorial team. And to all of the hard-working gang at the office, especially Paul Hunt, Louise Holland, Claire Postans, Zoe Collins, Sy Brighton and Ali Solway. To Tamsyn Zietsman, Laura Jones, Ben Lifton and the rest of the PR and marketing crew, and to the wider support teams – personal, operations, legal, finance, IT and, of course, my loyal army of office testers – I salute you!

On pictures, and there are a lot of snaps in this bad boy, big thank you to my dear friend David Loftus and his sidekick on lighting and digital, Richard Clatworthy. Thank you Dave, for going out of your comfort zone and embracing studio lighting on this one – I'm really happy with what we've achieved together. Shout out as well to my man Paul Stuart for the brilliant cover and portraits.

On design – and this one is clean, clear, bold and beautiful – massive thank you to James Verity at creative agency Superfantastic, and for your help on the book shoots, too (as well as indulging my requests for old-school indie tunes).

To the ever-supportive Penguin Random House posse, led into the fray by the don Tom Weldon and lovely Louise Moore. Special shout out to John Hamilton, Juliette Butler, Nick Lowndes, Elizabeth Smith, Merle Bennett, Clare Parker, Chantal Noel and Chris Turner, and to the wonderful gang making up their respective teams, Katherine Tibbals, Stuart Anderson, Jenny Platt, Anjali Nathani, Catherine Wood, Lucy Beresford-Knox, Celia Long, Martin Higgins, Katie Corcoran, Olivia Whitehead, Ben Hughes, Amy Wilkerson, Duncan Bruce, Samantha Fanaken and Jessica Sacco. And to the precious Annie Lee, Caroline Pretty and Caroline Wilding.

On to TV, and boy I'm excited about this series – massive shout out to the office team, and to all the crew that worked on the show. I have big appreciation for Katy Fryer, Sean Moxhay, Katie Millard, Ed St Giles, Niall Downing, Sam Beddoes, Gurvinder Singh, Leona Ekembe, Kirsten Hemingway, James Williams, Akaash Darji, James Bedwell, Kay Bennett, Mike Sarah, Joe Sarah, Dave Miller, Cliff Evans, Dave Minchin, Jim McLean, Jonnie Vacher, Calum Thomson, Luke Cardiff and Pete Bateson. Thanks to the guys that took care of the grub during filming – Krzysztof Adamek, Fred Augusts, Rogerio Nobrega and Ryan France. Big shout out as always to Lima O'Donnell, Julia Bell and Abbie Tyler, too.

Over at Channel 4, thanks to Jay Hunt, Sarah Lazenby and Kelly Webb-Lamb – thank you for believing in me and supporting my vision. Respect to the Fremantle team, too.

And, of course, last but by no means least, to my beautiful wife Jools, my band – Poppy, Daisy, Petal, Buddy and River – to Mum, Dad, Anna, Mrs N and Gennaro. Love you all X

Recipes marked   are suitable for vegetarians

316

For a quick reference list of all the dairy-free, gluten-free and vegan recipes in this book, please visit:

BOOKS BY JAMIE OLIVER

The Naked Chef 1999

The Return of the Naked Chef 2000

Happy Days with the Naked Chef 2001

Jamie's Kitchen 2002

Jamie's Dinners 2004

Jamie's Italy 2005

Cook with Jamie 2006

Jamie at Home 2007

Jamie's Ministry of Food 2008

Jamie's America 2009

Jamie Does . . . 2010

Jamie's 30-Minute Meals 2010

Jamie's Great Britain 2011

Jamie's 15-Minute Meals 2012

Save with Jamie 2013

Jamie's Comfort Food 2014

Everyday Super Food 2015

Super Food Family Classics 2016

Jamie Oliver's Christmas Cookbook 2016

5 Ingredients – Quick & Easy Food 2017

For handy nutrition advice, as well as videos, features, hints, tricks and tips on all sorts of different subjects, loads of brilliant recipes, plus much more, check out

JAMIEOLIVER.COM

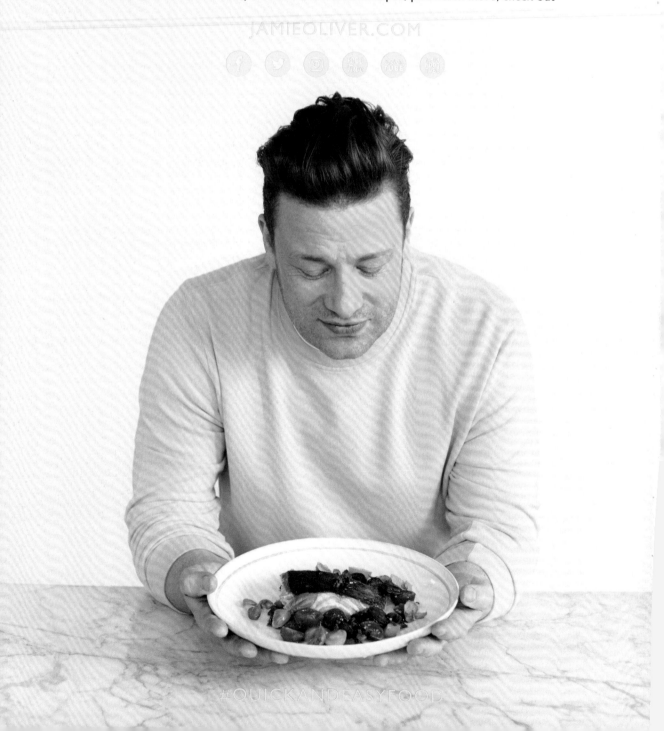

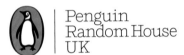

UK | USA | CANADA | IRELAND | AUSTRALIA | INDIA | NEW ZEALAND | SOUTH AFRICA

Michael Joseph is part of the Penguin Random House group of companies,
whose addresses can be found at global.penguinrandomhouse.com

Penguin
Random House
UK

First published 2017

031

Copyright © Jamie Oliver, 2017

Recipe and dedication page photography copyright © Jamie Oliver Enterprises Limited, 2017

Jacket and studio photography copyright © Paul Stuart, 2017

© 2007 P22 Underground Pro Demi, All Rights Reserved P22 type foundry, Inc.

Design by Superfantastic

Colour reproduction by Altaimage Ltd

Printed in Italy by Graphicom

A CIP catalogue record for this book is available from the British Library

ISBN: 978–0–718–18772–9

penguin.co.uk

jamieoliver.com

www.greenpenguin.co.uk

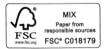

Penguin Random House is committed to a
sustainable future for our business, our readers
and our planet. This book is made from Forest
Stewardship Council® certified paper.